AF566823

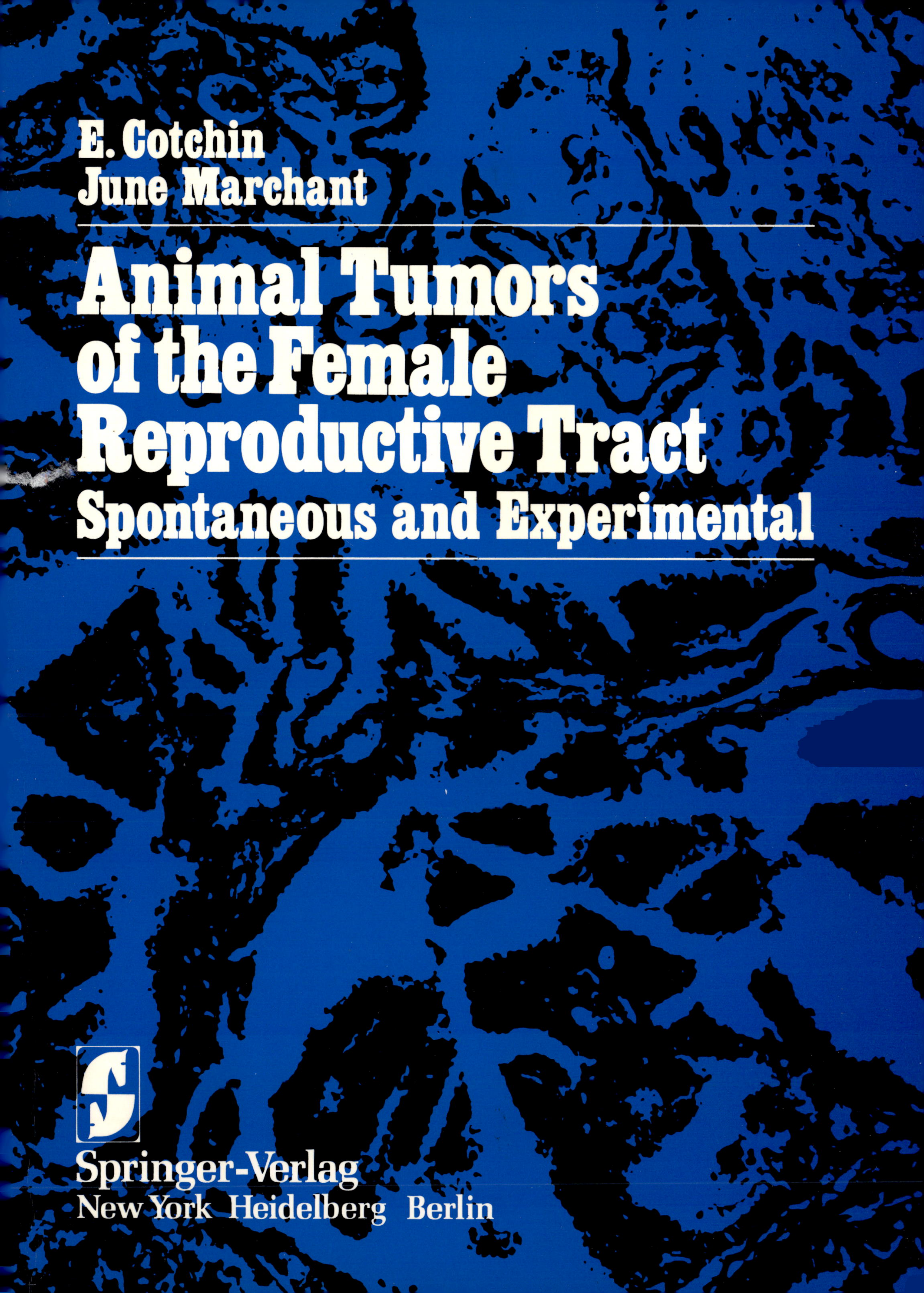
E. Cotchin
June Marchant
Animal Tumors of the Female Reproductive Tract
Spontaneous and Experimental
Springer-Verlag
New York Heidelberg Berlin

Animal Tumors of the Female Reproductive Tract

E. Cotchin
June Marchant

Animal Tumors of the Female Reproductive Tract: Spontaneous and Experimental

with 47 illustrations

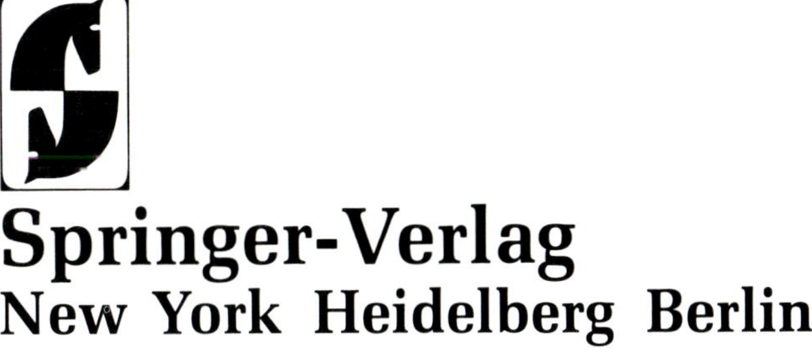

Springer-Verlag
New York Heidelberg Berlin

E. Cotchin, D.Sc., F.R.C.V.S., F.R.C. Path.
Department of Pathology
Royal Veterinary College
University of London
Camden Town
London NW1, OTU
England

June Marchant, Ph.D.
Senior Lecturer in the Biology of Cancer
Regional Cancer Registry
Queen Elizabeth Medical Centre
Birmingham B15 2TH
England

Special edition of Chapters 38 and 39 of *Pathology of the Female Genital Tract* edited by Ancel Blaustein, M.D.

Library of Congress Cataloging in Publication Data

Cotchin, Ernest.
Animal tumors of the female reproductive tract.

Bibliography: p.
Includes index.
1. Generative organs, Female—Cancer.
2. Oncology, Experimental. 3. Diseases—Animal models. I. Marchant, June, joint author. II. Title. [DNLM: 1. Animals, Laboratory. 2. Disease models, Animal. 3. Neoplasms, Experimental. 4. Ovarian neoplasms. 5. Uterine neoplasms. WP322 C843a]
RC280.G5C64 616.9'92'65 76-30730

Printed in the United States of America

ISBN 0-387-90209-0 Springer-Verlag New York
ISBN 0-540-90209-0 Springer-Verlag Berlin Heidelberg

Preface

The chapters which comprise this book were prepared as part of a medical text, *Pathology of the Female Genital Tract,* which is intended for the obstetrician, gynecologist, and medical pathologist. In that context, we were concerned to bring out the importance of the study of tumors of the female reproductive tract of animals, both as showing the variety of spontaneous neoplasms that might affect the tract and as providing tumors capable of experimental reproduction. These chapters are published separately, since they contain information which may appeal to a range of readers who might not necessarily wish to acquire the full medical text—for example, to veterinary and comparative pathologists, cancer research workers, research workers in gynecology, experimental pathologists and endocrinologists, and possibly to others using animals in experimental and pharmaceutical studies.

The survey of spontaneous tumors of the female reproductive tract is largely concerned with tumors of the ovaries and uterus of domesticated animals, but attention is also given to laboratory animals, wild animals, and animals in zoos. The spontaneous tumors are well worth studying, not only because of their obvious clinical importance to veterinarians, but also because they might provide a stimulus for epidemiologic, etiologic, biologic, and therapeutic investigations that may elucidate some of the problems related to their counterparts in humans. While some of these tumors are quite common, others are rare, and this negative kind of observation may be of great significance: for example, uterine cervical carcinoma and choriocarcinoma are, as judged from published accounts, practically confined to the human species. If this is confirmed, support will be gained for the proposition that factors more or less specific to the human patient may be involved in their causation.

The account of animal models has two aims. First, we show how the study of experimental tumors may throw light on the factors that may be of importance in producing tumors in humans, or indeed in other species. Second, we provide practical information for those workers who wish to undertake research on tumors of a particular site as to what are the most suitable laboratory animals, and which are the best methods for their purpose. The likely complexity of factors that may underlie the development of spontaneous tumors in humans and in animals is underlined by the observation that the same type of tumor has been shown to be capable of being induced experimentally by more than one type of carcinogenic agent. Again, the possible importance of intrinsic factors in tumor development is illustrated by the fact that the site and type of tumor induced in animals by any particular method may vary considerably according to the genotype of the animals used and to their age at exposure to the carcinogenic stimulus.

E. Cotchin
June Marchant

Contents

Preface

Chapter 1
Animal Models for Tumors of the Ovary and Uterus 1

General Introduction 1

Animal Models for Tumors of the Ovary 1

THE OVARY AS A TUMOR MODEL 2
Spontaneous Ovarian Tumors in Laboratory Animals 2
Methods of Inducing Ovarian Tumors in Mice 4
Direct Methods 4
X-Irradiation 4
Chemical Carcinogens 4
Transplantation 5
Ovarian Vasoligation 6
Thymectomy 6
Genetic Deletion 6
Indirect Methods 6
Intrasplenic Ovary Grafting to a Castrate 6
Parabiosis with a Castrate 7
Transplantation of a Gonadotropic Pituitary Tumor 7
Noncyclic Exposure to Bright Illumination 8
Chronic Exposure to Other Hormones 8

Progestational agents 8
Estrogens 8
Androgens 8
Thyroid hormone 8
Influence of Hormones on Ovarian Tumor Induction by Other Agents 8
PATHOLOGY AND HISTOGENESIS OF OVARIAN TUMORS 9
Tubular Adenoma 10
Granulosa–Theca Cell Tumors 10
Luteomas 10
Cystadenomas 11
Teratomas 11
Metastatic Tumors to the Ovary 11
ASSESSMENT OF THE PRESENT ANIMAL TUMOR MODELS OF OVARIAN CANCER 11

Animal Models for Tumors of the Uterine Fundus and Placenta 12

THE UTERUS AS A TUMOR MODEL 12
Spontaneous Uterine Tumors in Laboratory Animals 13
Methods of Inducing Tumors of the Uterine Fundus in Laboratory Animals 13
Hormone imbalance 13
Estrogens 13
Estrogens Plus Androgens 14
Progesterones 14
Testicular Grafts 14
Ovarian Fragmentation 14
Pituitary Growth Hormone 14
Carcinogens 14
Chemicals 14
3-METHYLCHOLANTHRENE (MC) 14
7,12-DIMETHYLBENZ[*a*]ANTHRACENE (DMBA) 15
2-FLUORENYLACETAMIDE (FAA) 15
N,*N*-FLUORENYLDIACETAMIDE 15
VINYL COPOLYMER 15
Intrauterine Devices 15
X-Irradiation 15
Viruses 15
Methods of Inducing Placental Tumors in Laboratory Animals 16
Chemical Carcinogens after Fetectomy 16
Virus after Fetectomy 16
Destruction of the Hypothalamic Nucleus 16

Animal Models for Tumors of the Uterine Cervix, Vagina, and Vulva 16
Methods of Inducing Tumors in Laboratory Animals 16
Hormones 16
Estrogens 16
Testosterone 17
Chemical Carcinogens 17
Dibenz[a·h]*anthracene (DBA) and Theelin* 17
Benzo[a]*pyrene (BP)* 17
3-Methylcholanthrene (MC) 18
Dimethylbenz[a]*anthracene (DMBA)* 18
Carbowax 1000 (Polyethylene Glycol) 19
N,N[1]-*Dimethyl*-N-*Nitrosourea* 19
Virus 19
Herpesvirus Type 2 (HSV-2) 19
ASSESSMENT OF THE ANIMAL TUMOR MODELS FOR CANCER OF THE UTERUS 20

Laboratory Animals as Hosts for Human Tumors 20

References 20

Chapter 2
Spontaneous Tumors of the Uterus and Ovaries in Animals 26

GENERAL INTRODUCTION 26
SPONTANEOUS TUMORS OF THE UTERUS 27
Domesticated Animals: General Survey 27
Mare (*Equus caballus*) 27
Ewe (*Ovis aries*) 27
Goat (*Capra hircus*) 28
Sow (*Sus scrofa*) 28
Dog (*Canis familiaris*) 28
Cat (*Felis catus*) 29
Fowl (*Gallus domesticus*) 29
Laboratory Animals: General Survey 29
Primates 29
Mouse 30
Rat 30
Guinea Pig 31
Hamster 31
Gerbil 31
Wild Animals, Animals in Zoos, and Birds: General Survey 31
Domesticated Animals: Detailed Account 32
Cow (*Bos taurus*) 32

Laboratory Animal: Detailed Account 34
Rabbit (*Oryctolagus cuniculus*) 34
SPONTANEOUS TUMORS OF THE OVARY 37
Domesticated Animals with Infrequently Reported Tumors 37
Ewe 37
Goat 37
Sow 37
Buffalo 38
Laboratory Animals 38
Primates 38
Mouse 38
Rat 39
Guinea Pig 39
Hamster 39
Gerbil 40
Ferret 40
Mastomys 40
Wild Animals, Animals in Zoos, and Birds 40
Insect Study 43
Domesticated Animals with Most Frequently Reported Tumors 43
Mare 43
Cow 44
Cat 47
Fowl 49
Dog 49
Types of Canine Ovarian Tumors 49
GROUP 1: PAPILLOMA AND ADENOMA 50
CARCINOMA 52
GROUP 2: GRANULOSA CELL TUMOR (GCT) 53
GROUP 3: SEMINOMA (DYSGERMINOMA) 55
TERATOMAS 56
General Discussion of Canine Ovarian Tumors 57
SUMMARY 60
References 60

Index 66

June Marchant, Ph.D.

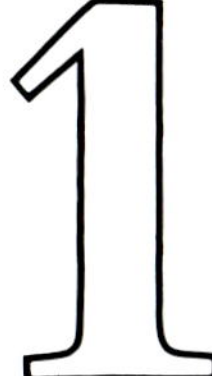

Animal Models for Tumors of the Ovary and Uterus

GENERAL INTRODUCTION

The ultimate objective of animal studies of cancer is to achieve a better understanding of factors responsible for human disease in the hope that this may be ultimately eliminated or controlled. In order to establish the basic biologic mechanisms governing the development of human cancer, systematic controlled experiments are required. For practical and ethical reasons, these are impossible to carry out with humans so animal models have to be sought.

Counterparts of many human diseases, including cancer, have been discovered occurring spontaneously in animals. Chapter 39 by E. Cotchin describes naturally occurring tumors of the ovary and uterus in many species. However, these examples are almost always sporadic and usually infrequent in their occurrence, and the most important requirements for cancer models in animals are that they be reproducible and predictable. They should also resemble the human counterpart.

ANIMAL MODELS FOR TUMORS OF THE OVARY

The first two requirements are best met by disease models that employ highly inbred strains of animals, such as the genetically pure lines of mice established many years ago by

C. C. Little and L. C. Strong by 20 consecutive brother–sister matings. Each pure strain has a different spectrum of spontaneous cancer incidence and different susceptibilities to cancer-inducing agents, as well as to other diseases. Since their pioneering work during the earlier part of this century, pure lines of other species of laboratory animals have been established and proved to be valuable tools in many studies, but the mouse and rat have been the most fully explored species with respect to tumorigenesis.

The third condition, that animal tumor models should resemble the human counterpart, is more difficult to achieve, partly because of the tremendous variation in the gross anatomy of the mammalian female genital tract. Some of these features are illustrated by Figure 38.1.

Comparing the human tract with that of common laboratory animals, one notices that human ovaries lie freely exposed to the general peritoneal cavity; in laboratory mammals, however, the ovaries lie in membranous pouches that partly (rabbit and guinea pig) or completely (rat and mouse) isolate them from the general peritoneal cavity. If the pouch (or bursa) is complete, the internal opening of the oviduct lies within it.[130]

Again, when we look at the uterus, the human species and higher primates have a "simplex" uterus with a single cervix. In the rabbit, however, the uterus is "duplex," having two long separate uterine horns with independent cervical openings into the vagina. Such a condition can occur as a structural anomaly in women on occasion.[63]

The cervix is defined[129] as the "caudal, nongestational portion of the mammalian uterus . . ." whose "epithelial lining is continuous with that of the vagina." The extent of this squamous epithelium into the uterine horns varies considerably in different species.

Another species variation is seen in the relative proportions, one to another, of the different parts of the female genital tract. These variations are matched by complementary variations in the anatomy of the penile structure of the male.[63] This lock and key principle is probably one of nature's ways of keeping different but closely related species distinct from one another.

This chapter considers first ovarian tumor models in laboratory animals. This is followed by animal tumor models of other parts of the female genital tract.

The Ovary as a Tumor Model

The ovary has many advantages as a model for disease. It is a well-defined entity that can be completely removed without the problem of residual rests. In the mouse, it is often small enough to be transplanted *in toto* back into the ovarian capsules from which it originated (orthotopic transplantation), or it can be exchanged for the ovary of another animal of the same genotype, or of another histocompatible genotype, with a high degree of functional success. With larger ovaries, vascularization of the complete organ is not achieved by this means; however, in such cases the organ can be cut into several fragments, and each fragment contains a full representation of all the different cell types present in the normal organ. Such fragments may be transplanted to a variety of different sites, including the anterior chamber of the eye, where they may become vascularized and remain under constant observation. Function of the transplant can be monitored by taking vaginal smears.

Of the thousands of oocytes present in the normal mouse ovary at birth, only a few are destined to be released during reproductive life. However, reduction in their number occurs by degeneration and this atresia continues throughout life. Its rate varies in different mouse strains and is particularly rapid in CBA mice, which develop a high incidence of spontaneous granulosa cell ovarian tumors in old age.[181] The rate of atresia is retarded when the pituitary is removed[82] and recent results have shown that it is speeded up by neonatal thymectomy, suggesting that a dual control mechanism may be controlling growth and maturation of follicles in postnatal ovarian development.[145] Atretic follicles in the stroma probably come to comprise the interstitial cells in the aging ovary, which are capable of responding to stimulation by pituitary hormones.

The number of oocytes present at birth in the ovaries of mice of different pure strains varies considerably.[83] Oocyte deficiency, which is the prime effect of aging, can lead to tumor development without further intervention, as will be seen later.

In the following pages, we shall examine the evidence in detail and see just how far the present tumor models of the mouse ovary, or the ovaries of other species of laboratory animals, can be made to satisfy the criteria of predictability, reproducibility, and resemblance to the human counterpart as an animal model of human ovarian cancer.

Because the literature is now very cumbersome, only key references are given. The reader desiring a more comprehensive reference list is referred to the excellent reviews by Jull[86] and Murphy.[137]

Spontaneous Ovarian Tumors in Laboratory Animals

The early report of Slye[174] on autopsies carried out on 22,000 mice suggested that tumors of the mouse ovary are quite uncommon. Only 46 solid ovarian tumors were

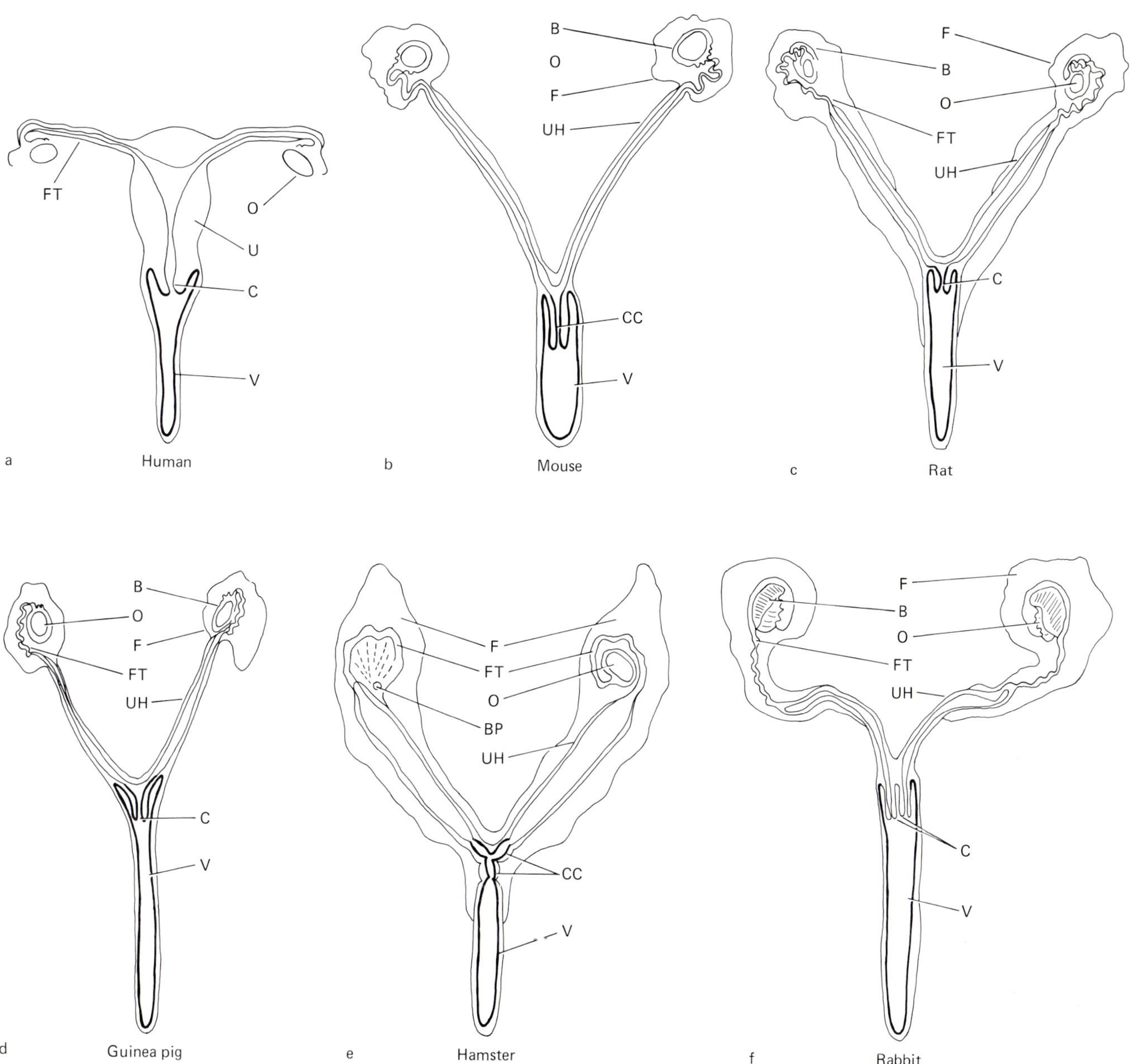

38.1 Comparative aspects of the female reproductive tract of the human and laboratory animal species. Redrawn and adapted from Hafez[64] and Mossman[130]. B, ovarian bursa; BP, blind pore; C, cervix; CC, cervical canal; F, fat; FT, fallopian tube; O, ovary; U, uterus; UH, uterine horn; and V, vagina. Note the complete (mouse and hamster), almost complete (rat, guinea pig), or partial (rabbit) enclosure of the ovary in a bursa, or pouch, whereas the human ovary remains free in the peritoneum. Also note the different proportions of the various anatomic sites, and the different extents of the vaginal squamous epithelium (heavy line) in the cervical region.

found, together with a small number of simple cysts. A recent report by Carter[19] on the autopsy records of approximately 3,000 female mice, mostly of random-bred Chester Beatty stock with a smaller number of Swiss albino mice and three inbred strains (BALB/c, CBA, and 101), revealed 18 ovarian tumors, only three of which were in untreated animals. He found only three ovarian tumors in 300 autopsies of female rats of the Chester Beatty stock (originally derived from Wistar animals). Reports of spontaneous ovarian tumors in guinea pigs and hamsters are rare and I have not found any report of them in rabbits. They have been reported in cats and monkeys and appear to be quite common in dogs and in fowl (see Chapter 39 by E. Cotchin).

Although it would seem from this that ovarian tumors are uncommon in rats and mice, they are seen much more frequently in research institutes holding certain inbred strains of mice if the animals are allowed to live out their normal life spans. They are not seen in some of the commonly kept strains, possibly because of the competing risks of other diseases; for example, in strains harboring the mammary tumor-inducing or leukemia-inducing viruses, death occurs from these causes at a much earlier age than is usually required for development of ovarian tumors in this species.

Many methods of inducing ovarian tumors in strains of mice in which they are not normally seen have been devised. They are of two types. There are those known as "direct" methods, which have an immediate deleterious effect on the ovary and can bring about tumorigenesis without further intervention. There are also "indirect" methods that do not have such a marked initial effect on the ovary but that bring about a chronic modification of its internal environment. I shall consider the different methods of tumor induction in mouse ovaries in turn and indicate which are applicable to other laboratory species.

Methods of Inducing Ovarian Tumors in Mice

Direct methods

X-IRRADIATION. This was the earliest discovered method of inducing ovarian tumors. It was first reported by Furth and Furth[42] that whole-body irradiation of mice with x rays could lead to ovarian tumorigenesis. It has since been confirmed by many investigators and is also an effective method in the rat.

The minimum dose required is around 25 R and the incidence rises with the dose received.[41] Administration of a single dose or chronic exposure to low dose levels, can be effective. By operating and drawing the ovaries out through a lead shield, it was shown that irradiation of the ovaries themselves was all that was required to induce tumors.[104] Conversely, irradiation of the whole body with the ovaries shielded induced no tumors.[28]

Work during the last decade has applied quantitative methods to show that irradiation has an acute effect on the mouse ovary, killing many oocytes within hours. After a dose of 25 R x rays given to 10-day-old mice, the residual oocytes were reduced to zero by the time the animals were 200 to 300 days old, whereas nonirradiated control animals still had several hundred remaining at 600 days.[149] At birth, mouse oocytes are very resistant to irradiation damage, but by 21 days their sensitivity is maximal. Thereafter they become more resistant.[154] At all ages, the smaller oocytes are more vulnerable.

The tumors induced by irradiation of the ovary of rats and mice are predominantly tubular adenomas.

CHEMICAL CARCINOGENS. To avoid confusing the reader with the former names of chemical carcinogens occurring in the older literature and their revised nomenclature, the key in Table 38.1 is appended for those most commonly used in this chapter.

7,12-Dimethylbenz[*a*]anthracene (DMBA) was the first chemical inducer of mouse ovarian tumors to be recognized. During investigations of mammary tumor induction in mice and rats with various polycyclic hydrocarbon carcinogens, a number of ovarian tumors were also noted in mice that had received DMBA in oily solutions painted on the skin.[73,120]

Since that time there have been many reports of ovarian tumor induction in mice by DMBA administered by a number of different routes: intragastric,[8] intraperitoneal,[96] intravenous,[101] subcutaneous,[172] direct application to the ovary,[97] neonatal injection,[172] as well as after brief *in vitro* exposure of the ovaries to DMBA, followed by reimplantation in the animals from which they had been removed.[87] There is evidence of a dose–response effect of DMBA *in vitro* as well as *in vivo*.[89]

Tumor induction time and incidence rates are influenced by age and strain of the treated mice.[115] Administration of DMBA to immature mice of two strains, induced tumors in all mice by 6 months.[96] Treatment of adult females gives a high incidence in mice of the C3H strain but not in the C57B1 strain.[101]

The experiments in which tumors have developed in reimplanted ovaries after exposure to DMBA *in vitro* suggest that DMBA itself is the effective carcinogen, rather than some metabolite formed by the liver,[89] and recent studies with tritiated DMBA also suggest this.[98] Nevertheless, when three of the metabolites of DMBA were tested, one of them was found to be effective *in vitro;* this was 12-hydroxymethyl-7-methylbenz[*a*]anthracene.[89]

It has also been shown that the related chemical, TMBA

Table 38.1 Chemical carcinogens

Symbol	Formerly called:	Now called:
BP	3,4-Benzpyrene	Benzo[*a*]pyrene
DBA	1,2,5,6-Dibenzanthracene	Dibenz[*a,h*]anthracene
DEN	Diethylnitrosamine	N-Nitrosodiethylamine
DMBA	9,10-Dimethyl-1,2-benzanthracene	7,12-Dimethylbenz[*a*] anthracene
FAA	2-Acetylaminofluorene	2-Fluorenylacetamide
MC	20-Methylcholanthrene	3-Methylcholanthrene

(7,8,12-trimethylbenz[*a*]anthracene) has ovarian tumor-inducing potential comparable with DMBA.[192]

Other polycyclic hydrocarbon carcinogens are relatively poor in inducing ovarian tumors in mice. 3-Methylcholanthrene (MC) is much less effective than DMBA[8] and I have seen very few ovarian tumors in many hundreds of mice treated with this carcinogen. Benzo[*a*]pyrene (BP) has only weakly carcinogenic action on the mouse ovary.[127]

In many experiments with these chemical carcinogens, particularly DMBA, there are competing risks of development of mammary tumors or leukemia, but if ovaries from a mouse treated with DMBA are grafted orthotopically to a new host of compatible genotype, or if ovaries are treated with DMBA *in vitro* and then reimplanted, only ovarian tumors are seen and the incidence may be virtually 100%.

Another chemical that can induce ovarian tumors in adult mice is the chemotherapeutic agent triethylene melamine, when injected intraperitoneally.[119]

A chemical method of inducing ovarian tumors that may prove to be very useful in future investigations is the intrauterine exposure of mice to urethane injected into the mother on days 11 and 13 of gestation.[147,197] Tumors induced by this treatment of ICR/J mice were cystadenomas. Ovarian teratomas have also been seen, whereas the vast majority of ovarian tumors induced in adult mice by chemicals are of the granulosa–theca cell series.

Rats respond to DMBA treatment in a different manner from mice. Although development of mammary tumors is frequently seen in both species, development of ovarian tumors does not occur in the rat. Instead, DMBA leads to severe adrenal necrosis in this species.[74] It has been shown that ^{14}C-DMBA is taken up in similar fashion by the adrenals and ovaries of both rats and mice,[88] so that different susceptibilities of the organs of the two species are not because of a particularly high ability to concentrate the carcinogen. It has, however, recently been shown that DMBA does have some tumorigenic potential for the rat ovary. Benign tumors arising in intrasplenic ovarian grafts in this species (see p. 6) become malignant and metastasize in many cases if DMBA treatment is also given. Treatment with a different potent carcinogen DEN (diethylnitrosamine, *N*-nitrosodiethylamine) had no such enhancing effect.[69]

Another chemical having some tumorigenic potential for the rat ovary is 2-acetylaminofluorene (2-fluorenylacetamide, FAA). In combination with the method of parabiosis (see p. 7), granulosa cell tumors were induced in 50% of the intact partners parabiosed to castrates and treated with FAA, whereas no tumors were found in untreated parabionts or in single females given FAA.[9]

An ovarian tumor has been reported arising in the offspring of a mother rat treated during pregnancy with FAA and progesterone. This tumor was classified as a "mucinous ovarian papillary adenocarcinoma." It was transplantable, had a short latent period of 14 days, caused ascites in 40 days, and killed in 60 days with metastases in lymph nodes, lung, and liver.[184] Benign mesovarial leiomyomas have been induced in Charles River CD rats by high and middle doses of mesuprine hydrochloride and soteronol hydrochloride, which are chemically similar and are long-acting, potent, β-adrenergic receptor stimulants.[142]

In guinea pigs and rabbits, DMBA does not give rise to ovarian tumors.[97] In Syrian hamsters, ovarian tumors have been seen after treatment with DMBA or MC, but the incidence is rather low.[70] Occasional tumors have also been seen in hamsters that have received BP or *o*-aminoazotoluene.

TRANSPLANTATION. Transplantation methods have been exploited in determining the function of different cell types of the ovary, and the relationships of the ovary with other organs have been explored by their use. Transplantation has also been much utilized in studying ovarian tumorigenesis in mice. Once a tumor-inducing method has been discovered, ovarian transplantation (for instance, from a treated animal to an untreated one and vice versa) makes it possible to separate the effects of the inducing agent into direct effects on the ovary itself and indirect effects mediated systemically through the host environment. Also, with the use of F_1 hybrids between two strains of differing susceptibilities to an inducing agent, transplantation methods facilitate studies of the factors determining the susceptibility of each of the genotypes.

Despite the advantages of transplantation in the above type of investigation, however, it cannot be regarded as an entirely innocuous procedure. When a mouse ovary is transplanted, even back into its own ovarian capsules, a large part of the tissue breaks down. If vascularization occurs, the grafted organ becomes reconstituted but never fully. There is an early decrease in the number of oocytes and ripening follicles that is associated with a shortening of reproductive life. The diminished amount of functional ovarian tissue may also lead to an imbalance of ovarian and pituitary hormones. Transplantation can, then, be regarded as a method of bringing about premature aging of the ovaries, resulting eventually in ovarian tumorigenesis.

It was observed that ovaries of DBA mice transplanted orthotopically into normal F_1 (DBA × C3H) mice became tumorous in five out of nine cases killed 12 to 24 months later.[75] Tumors have also developed in normal ovaries transplanted subcutaneously into castrated hosts of the same genotype.[86] Few tumors were seen if the hosts were ovariectomized females, but up to 80% were seen in some genotypes when the hosts were castrated males. These tumors were almost all tubular adenomas. If grafts came from DMBA-treated donors, however, tumors occurred in many of the castrated hosts of either sex, and they were predominantly of the granulosa–theca cell type.

In experiments with rats, ovarian fragments grafted into the anterior chamber of the eye of gonadectomized hosts all became vascularized after 1 year and many developed into granulosa cell tumors.[99]

OVARIAN VASOLIGATION. In the rat, abnormal ovarian activity can be brought about by ligating ovarian blood vessels temporarily. A continuous estrus is established, but it fails to control the hypophysis and the cytology becomes similar to that of a castrated animal.[35] A ligature of only 30 min was required to produce lasting changes, and ovarian tumors followed 20 months or more afterward.[36] This method of ovarian tumor induction does not seem to have been explored further.

THYMECTOMY. It has been shown, for three different mouse strains and four hybrid genotypes, that thymectomy before 4 days of age (but not at 7 days or later) leads to arrest in ovarian growth in approximately half of the females.[144] It was later observed that in two of the hybrid genotypes, thymectomized at 3 days and allowed to live their normal life spans, unilateral ovarian tumors of the granulosa or tubular adenomatous types developed in about half of them.[146]

There is also a mutant gene "nude" (nu) in mice, among the pleiotrophic effects of which are the absence of a thymus and infertility of both sexes.[151] These observations indicate a relationship between thymus and gonad during differentiation of the latter, which can be manipulated to give rise to ovarian tumors.

GENETIC DELETION. Among the mouse strains particularly susceptible to spontaneous ovarian tumor development are the CBA strain,[181] the CE strain,[29] C3H strain freed from mammary tumor-inducing virus,[27] RIII,[177] and various strains of New Zealand mice.[10] The incidence of ovarian tumors in females of these strains reaching an age of 18 months or more may be very high.

Mutant genes of the W series can lead to a high incidence of spontaneous ovarian tumors in mice carrying them.[139,165] The gonads of W^vW^v mice are deficient in oocytes at birth, because of a failure of the primordial germ cells to multiply between the eighth and twelfth days of fetal life. The animals are sterile and the females develop a 95% incidence of bilateral tubular adenomata of the ovary at about 7 months of age. F_1 hybrid (C57B1 × C3H) mice with W^xW^v genes develop tumors by 5 months and they have been shown to have significantly elevated levels (fourfold) of gonadotropins (both luteinizing and follicle stimulating hormones) during the pretumorous period.[140]

Genes of the steel (Sl) series have similar effects.[137] Some of the homozygotes are not viable, because of severe macrocytic anemia, but a high proportion of the less severely affected genotypes, such as Sl^d/Sl^d and Sl/Sl^d, survive to adulthood and develop ovarian tumors in old age.

These ovarian tumors of mice represent a constitutional disease dependent to a significant extent on genetic factors of two classes; there are those that result from the action of a single mutant gene, and those with polygenic inheritances that appear spontaneously with characteristic frequencies in different strains of mice.

The disadvantage of using as a model mice whose ovarian tumors arise from a single gene mutation is that these genes have pleiotropic effects. Animals carrying them also have defective hematopoiesis giving rise to macrocytic anemia, and they may not survive to the age when ovarian tumors may develop. Also, as a result of the ovarian dysgenesis, many of the genotypes carrying the mutant genes are sterile, so maintenance of the gene in the population requires complicated breeding programs.

Advantages of using a strain of animals in which the ovarian tumor susceptibility is determined by polygenic inheritance are that many of these strains are quite longlived and there are few problems about breeding them.

Indirect methods

INTRASPLENIC OVARY GRAFTING TO A CASTRATE. Ovaries transplanted to the spleens of castrated rats by Biskind and Biskind[12] were found to develop into tumors with great regularity. A similar operation in mice was soon shown to have the same effect.[43]

It had already been shown that subcutaneous implants of estrogen pellets in ovariectomized rats induced constant estrus, whereas intrasplenic pellets did not. It was postulated that tumors developing from the intrasplenic ovarian grafts resulted from hormonal imbalance; steroid hormones secreted from the grafts would be destroyed in the liver, just as the estrogen from the intrasplenic pellets, and thus rendered unable to exert their normal feedback inhibition of pituitary gonadotropins. These would be secreted chronically instead of cyclically, at an elevated level that would heighten the stimulation of the ovarian graft in the spleen, giving rise to hyperplasia and eventually neoplasia.

Support for this concept came when it was found that if one ovary remained *in situ* no ovarian tumors developed in the intrasplenic ovary[13] and, further, when it was shown that tumorigenesis could be inhibited by high systemic levels of estrogens or androgens, even when their administration was delayed for 3 or 4 months after transplantation.[103] Ovaries grafted into the pancreas were also found to become tumorous, demonstrating the significance of transplanting into the hepatic portal drainage system. Furthermore, repeated injections of luteotropin (LH) or of pregnant mare's serum were found to increase tumor incidence.[11]

In a recent experiment with rats, levels of both progestins and LH were measured and found to be high, and ovarian tumors developed in all animals bearing intrasplenic ovarian grafts without vascular adhesions. Hormone levels were much lower and no ovarian tumors appeared in such grafts if the animals were given an Eck fistula, which would produce hepatic bypass of the hormones from the intrasplenic ovaries by a portacaval shunt.[102]

Intrasplenic grafting of an ovary to a castrated rat or mouse leads to the appearance of benign "luteomas" after about 6 months, but granulosa cell tumors may appear in them later.[12] Early benign tumors may also be made to become malignant and to metastasize to the liver if DMBA treatment is also given.[68]

In rabbits with intrasplenic ovarian grafts, granulosa cell tumors have been seen after about 18 months.[152] In guinea pigs, large "luteomas" appeared in a similar length of time, but granulosa cell tumors were not seen before 5 years in this species.[121] In Golden hamsters, tumors do not develop in intrasplenic ovarian grafts.[93]

Parabiosis with a castrate. From what we have seen in the preceding section, one might expect that any way of achieving a persistently high level of gonadotropic hormones might act on residual ovarian tissue to give rise to hyperplasia and subsequent neoplasia in rats and mice and some other species. One method of achieving this is by parabiosis (suturing together side by side) of an intact female with a castrated partner. In this situation, excess gonadotropic hormones circulating in the castrate readily pass over into the circulation of the normal parabiont and stimulate its ovaries to produce larger amounts of estrogens, which are detectable by vaginal smears. However, when an attempt was made to induce ovarian tumors by this method in mice, the high estrogen levels reached, led to hydronephrosis and early death. In one pair that survived 9 months, an ovarian tumor was observed.[132]

Better survival occurs in parabiotic triplets with one intact partner joined to two castrated ones the same side. In this situation the estrogens passing from the normal partner are metabolized before they can reach the furthest castrate, whose pituitary remains stimulated. Excess gonadotropins produced by this partner are less readily metabolized than the estrogens, and they do reach the normal triplet in elevated amounts.

Parabiosis of an intact female mouse to one or two castrates has been shown to speed up the appearance of ovarian tumors induced by other methods. Induction time for ovarian tumors in irradiated mice has been reduced from around 24 months to 15 by parabiosis to a single castrated partner. It only slightly reduced the 10 months required for tumor induction by intrasplenic ovary grafting, but with two castrate partners, this was reduced to 5 to 6 months.[133]

I have already mentioned the synergistic effect of parabiosis to a castrate combined with administration of FAA in tumor induction in rat ovaries where neither agent alone was effective[9]. Parabiosis of a castrated male or female rat with a hypophysectomized female, a constant estrous female, or an intact male with a grafted ovary will also lead to ovarian tumors in this species.[81]

Transplantation of a gonadotropic pituitary tumor. It has been reported that transplants of a pituitary tumor secreting FSH and LH produced granulosa cell tumors of the ovary in eight of 146 female A × C rats at a much earlier age than have been the seven spontaneous tumors found in 1,812 old females of this same strain.

Two ovarian tumors so induced were transplanted and showed some degree of dependence on gonadotropins. These ovarian tumors in turn produced estrogenic effects (large uterus, pituitary, and mammary glands) as well as androgenic effects (enlarged clitoris and paraurethral glands). Pituitary hyperplasia led to excessive amounts of prolactin being produced which, together with estrogen from the ovarian tumors, stimulated the mammary glands to become neoplastic.[76] Mammary gland tumors were fast growing compared with ovarian and pituitary ones that preceded them, thus permitting the full chain reaction to occur in a single individual.

NONCYCLIC EXPOSURE TO BRIGHT ILLUMINATION. The incidence of tumors arising in rats with ovarian ligatures was enhanced in animals exposed continually to electric light[36] and 56 out of 60 rats exposed to continuous light from fluorescent lamps for 6 weeks showed persistent vaginal estrus.[173] There was progressive atrophy of the ovaries, which were full of cysts from tertiary follicles. These conditions were reversible and I am not aware of any experiments in which constant bright lighting alone has any tumorigenic effect on mammalian species. It has been observed that Brown Leghorn hens kept in a constant climatic chamber at a temperature of 65°F, relative humidity 60%, with 12 hr of fluorescent lighting but no natural daylight, had no annual cycle of egg laying. Egg production was continuous and gradually fell off over several years and hatchability declined. After 3.5 to 6.8 years, 19 out of 19 died and adenocarcinoma that involved the ovary, oviduct, mesentery, and intestine was seen. A control group in an intensive house, with 12-hr light in winter provided by a 100 W electric bulb, had the usual cyclic phase of molting and decline of egg laying in the winter months and only three developed adenocarcinoma and one a sarcoma in up to 12½ yr.[61] This suggests that under the conditions of bright lighting, without seasonal variation during the year, sustained gonadotropins are produced in these birds leading to the continuous egg-laying and subsequent sterility and neoplasia.

It would appear that in all the four methods of ovarian tumor induction outlined above, a constant elevated level of stimulation of the ovarian tissue by pituitary gonadotropins is being achieved and we must assume that this is the fundamental mechanism of tumorigenesis.

CHRONIC EXPOSURE TO OTHER HORMONES. Chronic exposure to a variety of hormones, both male and female, can lead to tumor induction in laboratory animals.

Progestational agents. During chronic treatment of mice with synthetic progestins used as contraceptive agents in women, it was noted that subcutaneous pellets of 19-norprogesterone led to ovarian tumors in four out of 18 BALB/C mice after 13 months or more.[109] A small incidence was seen after implantation of progesterone itself and in two of 24 mice that received norethynodrel (17-ethinyl-^{5,10}-19-nortestosterone); but ovarian tumors occurred in 13 out of 45 mice receiving implants of norethinodrone (17-ethinyl-19-nortestosterone).[106,108]

Estrogens. Chronic administration of estrogens to mice leads to hydronephrosis. Stilbestrol administered daily to rats leads to the development of huge cysts in the ovaries, filled with yellow caseous material, and to pyoovarium, pyometra, and uterine metaplasia.[64] In hamsters, chronic administration of estrogen leads to kidney tumors,[93] but in dogs, stilbestrol administration induces tumors of the ovary;[79] see Chapter 39 by E. Cotchin.

Androgens. Normal ovaries grafted subcutaneously or intratesticularly into male mice of the same genotype frequently develop into tumors, whereas subcutaneous grafts into intact females do not.[48] However, the rate of ovarian tumor induction is also high when ovaries are grafted to castrated males. When castrated animals of both sexes are compared, tumor induction occurs more frequently in castrated males than in castrated females.[85] These differences may be caused by sexual differentiation of the hypothalamus that occurs during the neonatal period in rats and mice, giving rise to a tonic (continuous) pattern of gonadotropin secretion in males and cyclic release in females.[57,155]

Administration of testosterone propionate daily to female rats from the age of 3 days to 21 months led to hypertrophy of the clitoris and development of three theca cell ovarian tumors in 10 animals surviving 16 months or more.[72]

Thyroid hormone. Thyroid function affects the incidence of tumors developing in ovarian intrasplenic grafts.[126] Addition of thyroid powder to the diet resulted in fewer tumors. Thyroid inhibition with thiouracil or limitation of food intake had no effect.

Recently, proliferative and neoplastic changes have been reported to occur in ovaries of hamsters treated with iodine-131 and methylthiouracil.[21]

INFLUENCE OF HORMONES ON OVARIAN TUMOR INDUCTION BY OTHER AGENTS. Not only does the administration of hormones lead to ovarian tumor induction in some circumstances, but changes in balance of ovarian hormones can also markedly affect ovarian tumor induction by other agents.

Ovaries from DMBA-treated mice will not grow into tumors in the absence of a pituitary in the host, although ovaries of hypophysectomized animals treated with DMBA will do so if transplanted orthotopically.[118] Development of tumors from DMBA-treated ovaries is therefore shown to be dependent on stimulation by pituitary secretions.

DMBA-treated ovaries grafted unilaterally to normal hosts will not develop into tumor,[117] nor will they if grafted subcutaneously to normal females. In the latter situation, removal of the host's own ovaries up to 6 months later will give rise to tumors in the DMBA-treated ovarian graft.[85]

Presence of a normal ovary also prevents tumor development from an irradiated ovary, as in the cases where only one

Table 38.2 Classification of spontaneous primary tumors reported in the human and other mammalian species[a]

Species	Total ovarian tumors classified	Cystadenoma	Carcinoma	Granulosa series	Dysgerminoma	Teratoma	Other	No. reports
Rodents (five species)	82	4	2	65	1	4	6	4
Guinea pig	3	0	0	1	0	2	0	2
Hamster	5	0	0	5	0	0	0	1
Equine	55	11	3	26	0	5	10	4
Sheep	1	0	0	0	0	1	0	1
Swine	31	11	3	4	2	2	9	4
Bovine	227	9	46	146	4	7	15	18
Feline	14	1	1	6	2	3	1	3
Canine	194	61	16	73	33	4	7	12
Monkey	13	4	1	3	0	2	3	2
All mammalian[b]	624	101 (16)	72 (12)	329 (52)	42 (7)	29 (5)	51 (8)	51
Human (two series)[b]	482	252 (52)	88 (18)	13 (3)	4 (1)	67 (14)	58 (12)	1

[a] Data condensed from Bonser and Jull.[14]

[b] Numbers in parentheses are percentages.

ovary has been irradiated,[104] and tumors do not appear in intrasplenic ovary grafts if one ovary is left *in situ*.[103]

The ability of ovarian hormones secreted from a normal ovary to prevent the emergence of ovarian tumors in situations where they would otherwise have arisen probably results from their control of pituitary gonadotropin secretion. However, it was not found possible to prevent development of granulosa cell tumors, in mice treated with DMBA, by periodic grafting of a normal ovary.[85] This may be explained by the fact that normal ovarian tissue grafted into intact female mice remains dormant and atrophic unless the host's own ovaries are removed. Normal ovarian grafts require deficiency of ovarian hormones in order to function, and DMBA-treated ovaries similarly require the same in order to develop into tumors. Some ovarian tumors themselves also have the same requirement and can grow only in ovariectomized hosts.

Exogenous administration of estrogens can inhibit tumorigenesis in mouse ovaries. No tumors developed in intrasplenic ovary grafts in castrated mice given regular injections of estradiol benzoate.[103] Injections of progesterone, in contrast, did not have any preventive effect at all.

The male environment has interesting effects on ovarian tumor development. Early observations of transplantable ovarian tumors in mice showed that these frequently grew better in intact males than in intact females. Tumor growth was also promoted by administration of testosterone to castrates.[134] Tumorigenesis was found to occur in subcutaneous grafts of normal ovaries to male mice of the same genotype and grafting to the intratesticular site was even more favorable.[46] Subcutaneous ovarian grafts in intact females, however, remain atrophic. When castrated hosts of both sexes were used, the castrated male environment was shown to be far more tumorigenic than the castrated female.[86] Despite the apparent tumor-favoring environment of the male animal, whether intact or castrated, administration of testosterone to mice bearing intrasplenic ovarian grafts inhibits tumorigenesis.[103] If delayed until 10 months after implantation, testosterone did not accelerate the growth of tumor nodules, which were already palpable. It was considered that any accelerating effect of testosterone on tumor growth was counteracted by its inhibiting effect on the pituitary gonadotropins required by the incipient tumors.[103]

Pathology and Histogenesis of Ovarian Tumors

The most common types of spontaneous ovarian tumors seen in rats and mice are tumors of the granulosa–theca cell series and tubular adenomas. Luteomas, teratomas, and papillary cystadenomas have also been reported but much more rarely.

In other nonhuman mammalian species, the commonest type of ovarian tumor seen is, again, the granulosa cell tumor. Table 38.2 summarizes the distribution of histologic types occurring spontaneously in the various species.

There appears to be no single mammalian species which resembles the human in its distribution of histologic types of ovarian tumor. In the human female, just over half of the ovarian tumors seen are primary epithelial tumors, whereas granulosa cell tumors comprise less than 10%. When all the other mammalian species are taken together, the proportions of these two tumor types are reversed.

Tumors induced in rats and mice by almost all the methods described are classifiable into tumors of the granulosa–theca cell series, luteomas, and tubular adenomas, with the first and last types predominating. Both the induction method and the genotype of the animal have some influence on which of the histologic types predominates.

TUBULAR ADENOMA. This is the most frequent type of tumor seen in mice after irradiation and in mice that have undergone genic deletion of oocytes. It is also the commonest type developing from normal ovaries transplanted into castrated male mice but is much less common in similar subcutaneous grafts in castrated females.[86]

Tubular adenomas are seldom seen after DMBA treatment and seldom arise in subcutaneous implants of ovaries from DMBA-treated donors in castrated hosts of either sex.[86]

Irradiated mice of the C57B1 strain develop tubular adenomas, whereas DBA mice give rise to granulosa cell tumors. "This indicates the importance of the genotype in determining the histology of the tumor."[131]

Tubular adenomas are usually bilateral and do not give evidence of hormonal activity. Transplants sometimes grow, although slowly, but they do so better in gonadectomized hosts.[6]

Tubular adenomas appear to arise from tubular downgrowths of the germinal epithelium that surrounds the ovary. The tubules gradually come to fill the ovary and there may be proliferation of interstitial cells among them that can become luteinized. This probably is the origin of some of the "luteomas" in the literature. Cells budding off from the linings of the tubules may assume the appearance of granulosa cells. Indeed, granulosa cell tumors and luteomas are sometimes a later development from tubular adenomas.

GRANULOSA–THECA CELL TUMORS. These tumors are the predominant type seen after DMBA treatment,[116] even when treated ovaries are residing in castrated male hosts, in which grafts of normal ovaries give rise to tubular adenomas.[86] They are also the commonest type seen in ovaries grafted to the spleen of castrated animals.

Again, certain genotypes are more susceptible than others to their induction, with IF, C3H, and DBA being particularly susceptible and C57B1 and BALB/c resistant. Grafts of ovaries from DMBA-treated females of the resistant strains will develop into granulosa cell tumors if implanted orthotopically in ovariectomized hybrid females[117] or subcutaneously in castrated males.[86] Resistance appears to be caused by a deficiency of pituitary stimulation that exists in the females of resistant strains, but not in the resistant males nor in females of F_1 hybrids between resistant and nonresistant strains.

Granulosa cell tumors are usually unilateral, with the ovary on the other side being atrophied. Evidence of secretion of ovarian hormones, such as enlargement of the uterus and constant estrus vaginal smears, is frequently present.

In the histogenesis of granulosa cell tumors after DMBA treatment, the initial event is one of oocyte destruction, with the oocytes of the smaller follicles being most susceptible.[97,116] This is followed by degeneration of granulosa cells and atresia of the follicles. When viable oocytes have gone, theca cells proliferate and undergo luteinization, becoming merged with remnants of old corpora lutea. This luteinized tissue may account for some of the "luteomas" described in the literature. Histogenesis of tumors in intrasplenic ovarian grafts is similar.[62]

Granulosa cell tumors are first recognized microscopically about 5 months after DMBA treatment, appearing as small nodules of basophilic-staining cells with densely stippled nuclei intermingled with acidophil luteinized cells. Tumor nodules are rarely seen in ovaries containing any viable follicles. It is considered that here "granulosa" cell tumor is a misnomer, because these tumors arise not from granulosa cells but probably from theca cells or other stromal elements.

Macroscopically, the early granulosa cell tumors present a pale pink appearance, but as they grow larger they may undergo considerable hemorrhage which gives them a dark purple cystic look. They may also show bright yellow areas of luteinization or be almost an entirely pale yellow.

If vaginal smears are followed during development of granulosa cell tumors following DMBA treatment, it is frequently found that estrous cycles gradually die out during the first months, giving a constant diestrous type of smear for a while. Later, animals usually go into a more or less constant estrus at the time when granulosa cell tumor nodules are first appearing.

Granulosa cell tumors are transplantable, but transplants grow slowly compared with most other types of mouse tumors and often show a preference for male hosts.

LUTEOMAS. Tumors composed of cells resembling those of corpora lutea are much less common in mice than the two previous histologic types mentioned, but they are seen in BALB/c × A F_1 mice after reimplantation of ovaries exposed to DMBA *in vitro*[87] and have also been seen after genic deletion of ovaries, x-irradiation, or intrasplenic grafting.

Transplantability is rare but it has been described.[44] The rareness may be because many of the "luteomas" described in the literature seem to represent a premalignant benign condition that precedes development of granulosa cell tumors, whereas "transplantable luteoma" may be a subsequent development of some granulosa cell tumors as they grow and mature.

Tumorigenesis appears to be much slowed down in castrated guinea pigs with intrasplenic ovarian grafts. These give rise to "luteomas" that may reach a size 50 to 100 times bigger than the normal ovary after about 2 years,[105] but they are not transplantable.[77] Only two granulosa cell tumors were seen in this species. These developed after nearly 5 years, and one metastasized to the liver.[121]

CYSTADENOMAS. Cystadenomas, one of the commonest primary epithelial types of ovarian tumor in the human species, have rarely been seen in animals, so the recent report of their induction in ovaries of ICR/Jcl mice is of great interest. Cystadenomas were seen in ovaries of mice whose mothers were injected with urethane on days 11 and 13 of gestation.[147]

TERATOMAS. Spontaneous ovarian teratomas in animals are extremely rare but they have been seen several times in C3H mice[189] and one of these was transplantable.[34] A case of bilateral teratomas was also seen in a Swiss albino mouse[33] and they have also been reported in CBA and DBA mouse strains.[123] These tumors also occur in *guinea pigs*[198,200] and have been reported in six ovaries from 1,176 female hares shot in New Zealand, where it is considered that DDT spraying may have been involved in their genesis.[38]

Recently a teratoma has been reported in a mouse exposed to urethane *in utero*.[148] Ovarian teratoma may also be induced to develop by parthenogenetically activating mouse eggs.[180] It is also of interest that testicular teratoma can be induced in mice of strain 129 by transplantation of 12½-day-old fetal gonadal ridges into adult testes,[179] from mouse egg cylinders,[24] or from displaced visceral yolk sac.[175]

METASTATIC TUMORS TO THE OVARY. The mouse ovary is a very frequent site for metastases from lymphomas. Tissue of the ovary may be almost completely replaced by lymphoma cells without apparent increase in size of the organ, which becomes smooth in outline.[119]

Assessment of the Present Animal Tumor Models of Ovarian Cancer

We are now in a position to assess whether the present animal tumor models of ovarian cancer make good models for the study of the human disease. The criteria we demanded of a good model were reproducibility, predictability, and resemblance to the human counterpart. How far do animal models of ovarian tumors satisfy these requirements?

There is no doubt at all that highly reproducible and predictable results can be achieved by many of the induction methods described. Some give tumors in virtually all of the animals that survive long enough to develop them, but it is important to avoid competing mortality risks associated with the inducing agent.

It is unfortunate that the most widely explored tumor-inducing agents have given rise to a distribution of histologic type of tumor quite different from the tumors appearing in the human species, although all the tumor types occurring in the human female have been seen developing spontaneously in animals. We have seen that tumors of different histologic types can be induced with a single technique by using mice of different genotypes or sexes. The development of these tumors is therefore probably a reflection of the differing hormonal environments acting on ovarian tissue at the time of action of the inducing agent. (I have personally seen a sequence of quite different histologic types of mammary tumors developing in C57B1 mice exposed to repeated DMBA treatment during the period when their immature ductlike "tree in winter" mammary tissue was being stimulated toward acinar differentiation by the progesterone of pseudopregnancy.) It is possible that deliberate focusing of direct tumor-inducing agents onto the ovary at different stages during its differentiation can yield a much greater variety of tumor types. Induction of cystadenomas and teratomas in recent experiments involving fetal or neonatal exposure to noxious agents or other manipulation seem to indicate that this may be so.

These considerations bring us to ask why the human species is apparently unique in its distribution of spontaneous ovarian tumor types.

The ovary is a highly specialized organ, an intricate complex of different cell types that has evolved from embryologic precursors. Possibly some of the precursors in the human ovary differ from those of other animals. It is of interest in this respect that a recent investigation using immunofluorescent techniques has shown specific intestinal antigenicity in the epithelium and mucin of human ovarian mucinous cystadenomas,[141] suggesting their frequent occurrence might be related to some occasional anomaly of ovarian development in the human fetus that leads to embryonic gut cells becoming incorporated in the developing organ. There they may lie undetected until influenced to undergo tumorigenesis, possibly by factors quite different from those giving rise to granulosa cell tumors of other mammalian species.

In contrast, recent induction of cystadenomas in mice by exposure of their mothers to urethane at a certain stage in their fetal development suggests that cystadenomas in human species result from exposure of the human fetus to some unrecognized environmental factor at a certain stage of gestation. Such a factor may be unrecognized because it may have no effect on tissues in later stages of differentiation.

We may also ask what the widely used animal models of ovarian tumors have taught us so far. They have emphasized the dominant role played by oocyte depletion (either induced or under genetic control) and the loss of follicles in the genesis of tumors of the granulosa–theca cell type. All the direct methods of ovarian tumor induction in mice (x-irradiation, chemical, transplantation, neonatal thymectomy, and genic deletion) bring about a premature loss of oocytes and follicles from the ovary. Tumors rarely appear before all viable follicles have gone. In the normal mouse (unlike the human female) oocyte depletion is not usually complete even at the end of the life span, which may be as much as $2\frac{1}{2}$ years. This may explain why spontaneous tumors are rarely seen except in mice of certain genotypes that lose their oocytes more rapidly than is usual.

Follicular disappearance would inevitably lead to changes in the normal cyclic levels of the pituitary gonadotropins, which would feed back in constant elevated amounts on the residual ovarian tissue deprived of its normal target tissue (normal ovarian follicle), stimulating it to hypertrophy and eventually to undergo neoplastic changes, as in the indirect methods of tumor induction (intrasplenic ovary grafting to a castrate, parabiosis to a castrate, transplantation of a gonadotropic pituitary tumor, noncyclic exposure to bright illumination, chronic exposure to steroid hormones).

Although it can be argued that such agents as irradiation and chemical carcinogens may cause mutations in certain ovarian cells that may later go on to form tumors, the apparent indefinite delay of their appearance by the presence of ovarian hormones in the host suggests that development of incipient tumors is completely dependent on continuing gonadotropic stimulation.

It can equally well be argued that continual hormonal stimulation of the ovary, such as is achieved by indirect methods of tumor induction, is the only essential factor in ovarian tumorigenesis in mice. The rodent ovary is, as Jull[86] said, "perhaps the best example of an organ in which hyperstimulation alone can cause tumorigenesis."

ANIMAL MODELS FOR TUMORS OF THE UTERINE FUNDUS AND PLACENTA

The Uterus as a Tumor Model

Cancer of the body of the uterus is one of the leading causes of female cancer mortality in developed countries and is geographically associated with various indicators of affluence. Cancer of the uterine cervix, which occurs in the region of the junction of the columnar epithelium of the uterine corpus with the squamous epithelium of the vagina, shows a quite different geographic distribution and is generally associated with low socioeconomic status.

It would seem, then, that cancer of the human uterine cervix and uterine corpus must be regarded as two quite distinct diseases with differing causative factors, and it is unfortunate that cancer mortality rates for some countries do not distinguish between them. In discussing tumor models, I shall endeavor to make the distinction but I shall include the vagina, which is lined by similar squamous epithelium, along with the cervix.

As explained in the introduction, the female genital tract of laboratory (and other) mammals is immensely variable in its gross anatomy and it must be borne in mind that the position of the squamocolumnar epithelial junction is also quite diverse. These factors, together with its much larger size, make the uterus a less convenient organ as a tumor model from the experimenter's point of view.

During the prenatal period, the human uterus undergoes a rapid spurt of growth during the last trimester, under the influence of maternal (possibly placental) hormones. Sudden removal of these hormones at birth causes very rapid involution of the organ during the first two postnatal weeks. These perinatal changes in growth rate occur mainly in the cervix, but the vagina shows similar changes.[25] At this early stage of life, therefore, the sensitivity of the cervix and vagina to female sex hormones is much greater than that of the uterine fundus.

Little attention has been paid to uterine growth in other fetal mammals, but it is known that in adult life there are definite cyclic changes in the histology of the cervix of the mouse,[58] rat,[65] and guinea pig.[90] In the absence of estrogen the transitional zone of the mouse resembles human metaplasia of columnar to stratified epithelium, but estrogen stimulation causes the transitional epithelium to disappear and an abrupt junction results. It seems that stratified epithelial cells of the transitional zone are very malleable and may differentiate to produce either keratinized cells or cells of a uterine type at the surface.[58] An early investigation in seven mouse strains also showed that, with advancing age, the processes sent down by the surface epithelium of vagina and cervix into the underlying connective tissue increased in depth, and this invagination was speeded up by estrogen injection.[182]

Similar changes also occur in rats. However, the vagina and cervix of the rabbit are lined at all stages with columnar epithelium that responds to estrogen by mucification, never by cornification.[25]

It appears, then, that the normal cervix is greatly influenced in its growth and differentiation by female sex hormones—much more so than the body of the uterus—and so it seems likely to respond in a more dramatic fashion to long-term imbalance of sex hormones.

Spontaneous Uterine Tumors in Laboratory Animals

As Cotchin has shown,[23] no animal species has yet been discovered with a significant incidence of spontaneous cancer of the cervix, suggesting that its common occurrence in women is caused by some specifically human factor.

Human endometrial cancer is less frequent than cancer of the cervix, the proportion being about 1:3 or 1:4 and the majority of patients being postmenopausal. Spontaneous endometrial cancer is uncommon in most animal species except monkeys, cows, and rabbits. These species are discussed in Chapter 39 by E. Cotchin.

In other laboratory species, spontaneous uterine tumors seem to be not infrequent in the rat, where 48 of 489 tumors were reported to be uterine,[18] and in the Golden hamster, where cervical carcinoma and adenocarcinoma, as well as uterine horn adenocarcinoma and leiomyosarcoma, have been seen.[162]

In the mouse, spontaneous tumors of the uterus and vagina are infrequent, except in certain strains and their hybrids. They were found in 13 of 56 exbreeding females of the Pybus Miller (PM) strain. Unfortunately this stock showed high sterility and was later lost. None were seen in six other stocks. Females of the PM strain often had imperforate vaginas and males had few mammary rudiments, suggesting a hormonal imbalance probably existed during fetal life.[51] Some uterine adenocarcinomas have also been seen in mice of the BALB/c strain, as well as in C3H females free from mammary tumor-inducing virus, and their first-generation hybrids. These tumors were transplantable.[30] Spontaneous papillomas and squamous carcinomata of the vulva have also been seen in mice of strain 129.[137] We see again the importance of genetic and hormonal factors in the etiology of these spontaneous female tumors of laboratory animals.

Methods of Inducing Tumors of the Uterine Fundus in Laboratory Animals

Hormone imbalance

ESTROGENS. In an early report, mice of the "Old Buffalo" strain given daily injections of estrogenic hormones (theelol and theelin) for 24 months developed proliferations in the uterus, cervix, and vagina that "in humans would have been considered malignant."[111] In most mice, however, the uterus responds to estrogen administration with hypertrophy leading to septic pyometra. Columnar epithelium of the uterine horns often undergoes squamous metaplasia or is replaced by extension of the squamous cervical epithelium. Carcinoma occurs only occasionally. However, tumors have occurred in high incidence in hybrid (PM × C3H) mice back crossed to PM, and in CBA mice and its hybrids treated with various estrogens.[50] Lesions were adenomas or adenocarcinomas, as well as infiltrative uterocervical epidermoid lesions, some of which were considered to be carcinomas. Hybrid (BALB/c × C3H) mice have given a similar range of tumors after injection of estradiol benzoate.[7]

Rat uteri respond to estrogens in a similar manner to most strains of mice, showing cystic hyperplasia, squamous metaplasia, and sometimes pyometra. Occasional tumors occur but spontaneous ones are not infrequent in this species.[3]

In guinea pigs, prolonged treatment with estrogen injections beginning early in life caused cystic glandular hyperplasia of uterine endometrium in every animal receiving more than 35 days of treatment. At first it was confined to the uterine horns; then it spread to the upper part of the fundus, the cells of which were swollen with glycogen instead of flat as in the cornua. Fibromyomas were seen after 200 days of treatment.[143]

Fibromyomatas were also induced at various other abdominal sites, such as pancreas, kidney, and spleen, by administration of all natural estrogens and by artificial ones. They occurred in castrated females and in intact or castrated males given larger doses. Some of the abdominal tumors invaded liver, pancreas, and muscle but not kidney and spleen. When the estrogen stimulus was withdrawn, they began to regress, undergoing hyalinization and ossification.[110] Spontaneous fibromyomas of women have a much more ordered arrangement of fibrous tissue than does myomata of the guinea pig.

In rabbits, some malignant growths have been described after administration of estrogens.[158] The high incidence of cystic endometrial hyperplasia and uterine tumors seen in old breeding females of some colonies after toxemia of pregnancy is believed to be caused by an excessive concentration of estrogen, resulting from impairment of liver function.[60]

When stilbestrol was given to rabbits with alloxan-induced diabetes, there was no enhancement of the stilbestrol-induced effect, although alloxan on its own produced endometrial hyperplasia and adenomyosis.[125] Examination of the endocrine organs led to the conclusions that estrogen had both direct uterine effects and indirect effects mediated through stimulation of the pituitary basophils and consequent ovarian stimulation. Cancerous animals showed hypertrophy of pituitary, adrenals, and ovaries, with indications of adrenocortical hyperactivity.[176]

Prolonged treatment of 10 squirrel monkeys with diethylstilbestrol led to malignant uterine mesotheliomas, originating from the serosa and presenting sometimes as solid sheets and sometimes in glandular or papillary form, in seven of the treated animals; the other three showed early lesions of the serosa.[122] This would seem to be a species with uteri particularly sensitive to tumor induction by estrogen.

Estrogens plus androgens. In all female Syrian hamsters given pellets containing both diethylstilbestrol and testosterone propionate, cystic glandular hyperplasia of the uteri occurred and there were multiple foci of nodular hyperplasia in the muscle of both horns. In addition, six out of 10 had multiple leiomyomas in one or both uterine horns that were indistinguishable histologically from the leiomyomas of the epididymes seen in five out of 11 males similarly treated.[5] Hormone dependency and progress toward autonomy following serial transplantation of similarly induced tumors has been demonstrated.[94]

Progesterones. In an investigation of progesterone and 19-nor-contraceptives in mice, tumors of the endometrial stroma, varying between fibrosarcoma and sarcoma, were produced by progesterone and norethindrone. Another 19-nor-contraceptive, norethynodrel, produced metaplasia of the endometrium and glandular epithelium.[107]

Testicular grafts. Leiomyomas arose in female rats that had received testicular grafts (usually two) from littermates when newborn. By sexual maturity, most animals had constant estrus, and pyometra began after 6 months. The uterus usually ulcerated into the body cavity through the digestive tract, or through the body wall to the exterior, and the animals died. Only 16 of 185 survived more than 3 years and four of these had uterine leiomyomas similar to fibromyomas that frequently occur in women.[156] One rat showing continuous estrus died at 2¼ years with a huge typical adenocarcinoma in the left uterine horn and numerous metastases. The pituitary of this animal was enlarged and hemorrhagic.[157]

Ovarian fragmentation. About 40 years ago, Lipschutz[105] and his colleagues showed that uterine tumors could be induced in guinea pigs by long-term results of subtotal castration, or "ovarian fragmentation" as he called it. One ovary was completely removed and only a fragment of the other left behind. An irregular sexual cycle reestablished itself with prolonged estrous and diestrous phases. The uterus, sometimes increased up to 10- or even 20-fold its normal weight, showed cystic glandular hyperplasia and metaplasia of the endometrium, as well as polyps filling the uterine cavity. Uterine glands were frequently seen in the myometrium, where some animals showed subserous adenofibromyomas. After 3 years or so, multifocal adenocarcinomas were seen in the small number of survivors.[105] As with prolonged estrogen treatment, other abdominal fibroids were seen. There was also nodular hyperplasia of the adrenal cortex, and a Brenner-type ovarian tumor occurred in one instance. The ovarian fragment contained lutein cysts, sometimes blood filled, and hemorrhagic follicles.[17] These observations and other experimental evidence led to the assumption that the ovarian remnant lost the faculty to control the gonadotropic function of the hypophysis.

Pituitary growth hormone. Daily intraperitoneal injections of pituitary growth hormone in gradually increasing doses gave hypertrophy of the myometrium in all 15 Long Evans rats and glandular cystic hyperplasia in two (one with a polyp). In one animal the entire right horn of the uterus was replaced by a tumor that adhered to the bowel and infiltrated the myometrium extensively.[128]

Carcinogens

Chemicals. *3-Methylcholanthrene* (*MC*). Large tumors of the mouse uterus have been induced by implantation of MC crystals, 1% MC in lard, or 1% MC plus 1% estradiol propionate. The mice used were CBA strain or outbred white animals. The implant was secured in place by ligatures above and below. In all, 14 out of 109 developed fibromyosarcomas, which were mostly locally invasive and tended to appear earliest. Twenty out of 109 developed endometrial carcinomas, which were more prevalent in the CBA strain. Immature CBA mice were particularly susceptible to uterine tumor development (12 out of 15).[15]

Another method that has been used to follow early stages in development of adenocarcinoma in the mouse uterus involves using cotton thread, part of which is impregnated with a 1:3 mixture of MC with beeswax. At laparotomy, the thread was inserted with a needle through the lateral wall of one uterine horn and pulled through the tip until the impregnated part lay in contact with the endometrium. Endometrial hyperplasia appeared after 7 weeks and there was fibrous proliferation of stromal tissue. A total of 32 out of 110 mice of the na 2 strain developed adenocarcinoma of the endometrium, three adenoacanthoma, two sarcoma, and two squamous cell carcinoma.[187] This method has been used to study enzyme histochemistry of the lesions.[188]

Tampons of cotton tape or silk strings impregnated with MC in polyvinylchloride and melted paraffin wax induced adenocarcinomas in rabbit uteri and squamous cell carcinoma in mice and rats.[3]

Homburger,[70] reviewing chemical carcinogenesis in Syrian hamsters, reported that in 161 female survivors (of seven different strains) given MC by stomach tube, there were 55 uterine tumors and 82 ovarian and 123 mammary tumors.

7,12-Dimethylbenz[a]anthracene (DMBA). In mice, as we have shown earlier in this chapter, DMBA leads to ovarian and breast tumors. In rats, administration of DMBA during early life (fetal, newborn, or 10 days old) to females of a Sprague–Dawley strain resulted in uterine tumors developing over 12 months in 13 out of 31 animals; six were adenocarcinoma, two squamous cell carcinoma, two myosarcoma, one anaplastic, and two mixed. Two metastasized to the lungs and abdominal viscera.[167] One uterine adenocarcinoma that was transplanted had metastases to the lungs when the hosts were injected with medroxyprogesterone acetate.[168]

2-Fluorenylacetamide (FAA). Rats of the Buffalo strain given FAA mixed in powdered food for a year, on the average, developed uterine fibrosarcomas in three instances.[183]

N,N-Fluorenyldiacetamide. In 10 spayed female A × C rats, this chemical induced cystic hyperplasia of the uterus and three sarcomas. Norethandrolone (17-ethyl-19-nortestosterone) caused endometrial cystic hyperplasia when administered alone, but when administered together with *N,N*-fluorenyldiacetamide it led to endometrial sarcomas (possible leiomyosarcomas). They did not appear in intact females so treated. Carcinosarcomas of the salivary glands also developed and had the same induction requirements.[161]

Vinyl copolymer. Cotton tampons coated with vinyl copolymer and paraffin wax melted together in a dish and inserted in one uterine horn of MIH Black rats induced marked inflammation of the endometrium and moderate enlargement with pyometra after 4 to 10 months and marked epithelial dysplasia at 10 to 12 months; at 10 to 18 months five out of 12 had squamous cell carcinoma. Controls with strings coated only with paraffin had similar changes, resulting in epithelial dysplasia at 18 months. One leiomyosarcoma was found but no carcinoma.

Tumors seen with the polymer strings were identical in ultrastructure to those seen with strings coated with MC, but the latent period of tumor induction was much longer with the polymer.[4]

INTRAUTERINE DEVICES. In experiments with virgin female Wistar rats, stainless steel or polyethylene loops or springs were sterilized and inserted in both horns of the uterus through a small incision and anchored with silk. After 14 months a sarcoma with widespread metastases throughout the abdomen appeared and after 19 months, when 19 were still alive, six epidermoid cancers appeared in the animals with the stainless steel devices.

With polyethylene devices, the first epidermoid carcinoma appeared at 20 months and a sarcoma occurred at 23 months. Epidermoid carcinomas were considered to be a rare feature in this rat strain.[22]

X-IRRADIATION. In rabbits, where uterine tumors are common in old animals, chronic exposure to low doses (8.8 R) of γ rays induced them in a much shorter period of time.[113]

Implantation of ^{60}Co wires in the pelvis of female rats for periods from 10 to 200 days induced adenocarcinoma of the uterus in 14 out of 32 females. The tumors were composed of dilated glands with scanty stroma, usually, and the longer exposures gave increased numbers of tumors. It was calculated that the uterus received approximately 16,000 to 961,000 rads, most of these doses being much too high to induce tumors in the ovary, which was often reduced to scar tissue.[71]

VIRUSES. Eight endometrial sarcomas and one leiomyosarcoma were seen to develop in 37% of F_1 (C57B1 × DBA) female mice reaching 18 months old or more. They were readily transplantable but did not respond to endogenous or exogenous progesterone; seven of these eight mice had been inoculated with either Friend or Rauscher leukemia virus.[26]

Methods of Inducing Placental Tumors in Laboratory Animals

Chemical carcinogens after fetectomy

Malignant tumors of placental origin have been induced in rats, guinea pigs, and rabbits during the past decade. Long Evans rats were mated and the females were fetectomized at 10 to 12 days. Beeswax pellets containing DMBA were placed in the gestation sacs of 144 animals (1,042 sacs). Most of them were also injected with Depo-Provera (medroxyprogesterone acetate) and they were killed at intervals from 7 to 40 weeks later. Sixty-five developed malignant tumors after 12 to 13 weeks, seven of which were choriocarcinomas. Three had pulmonary metastases. Many of the remaining tumors were adenocarcinomas of the endometrium and malignant mesotheliomas.[171]

Tumors histologically resembling human chorioadenoma destruens have been induced in Japanese Hartley guinea pigs following fetectomy at 4 to 5 weeks gestation. The placental mass was left *in situ* and a suspension of *N*-butyl-*N*-nitrosurea in carboxymethyl cellulose instilled into the uterus. Some of the animals received intramuscular injections of human chorionic gonadotropin as well. The tumors were quite proliferative, were composed of bizarre tumor cells that invaded the myometrium, and were seen also as perivascular infiltrates. Pleiomorphic cells resembled malignant cytotrophoblasts. The changes were much more striking in animals not treated with HCG.[170] However, the series is small and the effects of HCG are not certain. The small number was related to the fact that the guinea pig is prone to postoperative infection and only five of the 20 animals survived the procedure.

Virus after fetectomy

Choriocarcinomas have been induced in Wistar rats after fetectomy at 12 days of gestation and injection of Moloney's mouse sarcoma virus (MSV) followed by Depo-Provera on days 14 and 28. In most animals the injections were made into the placenta, but others were injected intravenously (i.v.) or intraperitoneally (i.p.). Control animals were nonpregnant, with MSV in one horn and control fluid in the other, both ligatured at the bottom to retain the fluid. No tumors were found in controls, but they were seen in 10 out of 29 rats injected with virus *in utero* and in two out of 10 injected i.v. or i.p.[193] Infectious virus could not be isolated from tumor cells, but the presence of the MSV genome could be demonstrated by a direct rescue test. Cytologic appearance supported the yolk sac origin of the tumors.

Destruction of the hypothalamic nucleus

Tumors resembling human choriocarcinoma were induced in two out of 15 pregnant rabbits after destruction of the hypothalamic nucleus by means of electrocoagulation. Coagulation was carried out at 8 to 14 days postcopulation. Fifty-five animals were treated; 10 died rapidly and 30 failed to show pregnancy. The two successful cases of induction had been treated on the ninth day (just prior to completion of the placenta). No macroscopic metastases were seen, but vascular tumor emboli were seen in the lungs of one of the two animals. No such tumors had been seen in 1,000 pregnant rabbits used for experiments during the previous 10 years.[100]

ANIMAL MODELS FOR TUMORS OF THE UTERINE CERVIX, VAGINA, AND VULVA

Methods of Inducing Tumors in Laboratory Animals

Hormones

ESTROGENS. In a series of publications dating from 1936 to 1959, Gardner and co-workers showed that mouse uterine reactions to high doses of injected estrogens varied markedly according to age. After weaning, estrogen results in hypertrophy of the uterus and pyometria. After birth, the entire uterine epithelium becomes stratified (but not cornified), with metaplasia extending into the uterine ends of the fallopian tubes. The vagina becomes greatly enlarged with increased thickness of the stroma caused by mucoid change.[49] Weekly injections of estrogens, continued for over a year, led to carcinoma of the cervix in 50 to 60%.[1] Mice of all strains responded in this way if they survived long enough, the highest tumor incidence occurring at 450 to 600 days. After cornification, the epithelium might atrophy before the earliest invasive lesions were seen. Grossly the cervices were firm and white with deficient blood supply.[45]

Cervical and vaginal tumors could also be induced in adult mice by pellets of stilbestrol–cholesterol attached to nylon threads, dipped in collodion, and placed in the vagina. They were also seen in some mice after intravaginal instillation of stilbestrol, three times weekly. Several mouse strains were used. Some did not tolerate the treatment well, but epidermoid carcinomas appeared in eight out of 40 BC mice with stilbestrol pellets and another 12 had smaller lesions after 260 days. Estradiol benzoate administered weekly was also effective, and addition of testosterone to estrogen–cholesterol pellets did not diminish the incidence. Other substances under consideration for use in intravaginal contraceptives (urea, adipic acid, and carboxymethyl cellulose) also induced invasive lesions of the vagina after 500 days or more.[47]

Experiments by Dunn confirmed the effectiveness of estrogens administered on the day of birth. Injections of diethylstilbestrol in three mouse strains led to the formation of astonishing concretions in the vagina in 12 out of 30 after 13 months, as well as carcinoma of the cervix and vagina.[32] The antifertility drug Enovid, administered in liquid diet to newborn BALB/c mice, produced similar endometrial changes to estrogens, and some animals continued on Enovid for around 2 years, had lesions of the cervix diagnosed as early cancer.[31] These findings preceded the report that large doses of stilbestrol, given to pregnant women with threatened abortion, could lead to adenocarcinoma of the vagina developing in their daughters 14 to 22 years later.[66]

The early changes seen after treatment of newborn mice with estrogens have been studied and found to be greater with diethylstilbestrol than with the same dose of estradiol.[39] They are not abolished by ovariectomy with or without adrenalectomy or hypophysectomy. Vaginal epithelium continued to proliferate and cornify after transplantation into ovariectomized hosts and frequently showed hyperplastic lesions of the epithelium that occasionally transformed into carcinoma-like tumors after 6 months. Serial transplantation of such vaginas under the abdominal skin of ovariectomized females may result in malignancy, and metastatic cancer has been seen in two instances after the fourth transplant.[186]

Testosterone. Subcutaneous implants of testosterone pellets twice a week in female (C57Bl × DBA) mice starting at 6 to 13 weeks old induced uterine tumors in 26 out of 42 in 15 to 18 months, mostly in the cervix or unpaired uterine part. Histologically there were large trabeculae of cells next to solid nests; they formed locally branched papillae inside large sinuses, and most infiltrated the uterine wall. Mice without gross tumors had pink nodules of similar tissue in the stroma of the endometrium. These growths resembled the histologic changes seen in the endometrial stroma during early pregnancy and the hypothesis was advanced that the tumors were related to decidua cells.[194] Many extended into muscle of the uterine wall and some also had lung metastases. Transplants of two tumors grew in androgen castrates, but not in untreated castrates, showing that they were androgen dependent. One of these became autonomous and caused marked atrophy of the ovaries when grafted to intact females.[195]

In another investigation, female BALB/c mice treated neonatally with estrogen or testosterone propionate (at dose levels associated with the induction of persistent vaginal cornification) showed hyperplastic lesions of the vagina resembling epidermoid carcinoma (15 to 17 months later after either hormone). These lesions were reduced in incidence in animals that were ovariectomized around 4 months of age, and there were dose-dependent effects on the epidermization of the middle region of the uterine horns.[92]

Chemical carcinogens

Dibenz[*a* · *h*]anthracene (DBA) and theelin. One of the earliest studies in the induction of cancer of the cervix used unpedigreed adolescent female mice, half of which were spayed. Their skin was painted twice a week with DBA solution in benzene and half of each group were also later treated with theelin. Among the great variety of tumors arising was epidermoid cancer of the cervix in three animals that had received treatment with both agents and carcinoma of the uterus and vagina in two that had received similar treatment.[153] These early experiments were soon followed by others using different polycyclic hydrocarbon carcinogens.

Benzo[*a*]pyrene (BP). When BP in cholesterol was broken into fragments of about 5 mg and placed into the vagina of 10 mice two or three times a week, tumors appeared in all after 10 to 14 months. They were first seen on the vaginal wall and all were infiltrating squamous cell carcinoma.[37] Similar applications of human smegma from elderly institutionalized men was quite ineffective.

Other methods of applying carcinogens were devised, such as painting acetone solutions on the cervix with cotton-tipped wire loops,[199] later aided by the use of an infant-sized otic speculum,[95] or by impregnating strings that were then threaded into place and secured with knots or stitches at laparotomy.[78] Most experiments with BP, however, have used the direct painting method, and this model has been used to study enzyme histochemistry of changes in the upper vagina,[191] for studies of histogenesis of cervical carcinoma,[163] and for autoradiographic studies of early atypic changes.[164]

All mice treated with BP directly in the vagina develop atypical changes that lead to cancer developing in those surviving long enough. The incidence of cancer induced by this method is high.

Rats appear to be less susceptible than mice to cervical tumor induction by BP painting of the cervix.[178]

3-METHYLCHOLANTHRENE (MC). This carcinogen was shown to induce cervical carcinoma when uteri of young female mice were removed, MC crystals were inserted, and the uterus transplanted subcutaneously on the upper abdomen of hosts (usually brothers or sisters) of the same strain. Of 104 mice of various genetic types, 55 developed 61 tumors (32 carcinomas and 29 sarcomas), the majority appearing by the eighth week. The A strain gave the highest incidence (21 tumors in 16 of 20 mice treated). More tumors occurred in the cervix than in the uterine horns and the tumors included epidermoid carcinoma, adenocarcinoma, adenoacanthoma, and sarcoma.[150]

An investigation using threads with three knots impregnated with MC in beeswax 1:3 and suspended in the vagina of C3H mice led to malignant neoplasms of the cervix developing from 7 weeks onward in the majority of animals. In all the animals with carcinoma, the cervix was involved and there were extensions of tumor into the uterus and upper vagina. A few showed metastases to paraaortic lymph nodes, and adrenal and lung were involved in one case each.[159]

In a review of the subject in 1957, a comparison was made of the string and painting methods with MC and BP in C3H female mice. The highest incidence of cervical tumors was obtained at 11 to 33 weeks by MC and the string method (85%). Then, in order, came BP string, MC painting, and BP painting (50%).[166] With the string method, most tumors were induced in the cervix, but painting gave many vaginal lesions. Many tumors were invasive and extended to pelvic nodes, with metastases seen in lung and liver. It was considered that the mouse anatomy was such that neither method would reach the high site of transition from squamous to columnar epithelium; nevertheless the lesions showed a striking resemblance to human cervical cancer.

MC painting of the cervix of mice has been used to show the evolution of dysplasia of the cervix and vagina.[201] An increased effect of MC on the uterus of spayed females was seen when estrogens were present, and lesser penetration of the stroma was seen if progesterone was injected in addition to estrogen.[91] More recent experiments showed that when progesterone was given in addition to MC treatment of the cervix, the tumors were significantly increased in number, giving a mucoepidermoid type of invasive carcinoma in the endocervix but having no maturational effect on tumors of the exocervix or vagina.[160]

Limited exposure to MC-impregnated threads gave increasing numbers of tumors as exposure increased from 2 to 4 weeks, and the addition of a diethylstilbestrol (DES) pellet increased the incidence. There were strain variations in susceptibility to both MC and DES effects.[136] Castration after-exposure to MC threads (knotted or unknotted to give high or low doses) markedly decreased the incidence of invasive cervical carcinoma (from 100 to 62% in A strain mice after a high dose of MC), thus showing the promoting effect of estrogen on cervical cancer.[138] This model has also been used to show the relationship of carcinogenesis with epidermization (spread of benign stratified squamous epithelium within the uterus),[59] as well as the histochemistry of the cervical epithelium during carcinogenesis,[114] the effect of anticancer drugs,[185] and the effect of neonatal treatment with estradiol on cervical carcinoma induction.[40]

The MC string method has also been used to induce carcinoma of the cervix in rabbits and here it seems to be uninfluenced by the addition of estradiol or progesterone.[2]

DIMETHYLBENZ[*a*]ANTHRACENE (DMBA). DMBA was first used by the knotted string method to induce carcinoma of the cervix in rats.[196] Eleven of 39 female Wistar rats surviving the operation developed gross tumors and two more had microtumors. Sometimes invasion into parametrial and endocervical tissue was detected, but no metastases were seen. The endocervix of 12 out of 13 rats with neoplasia was dilated and filled with keratin. In the walls, papillomas formed that ultimately transformed to epidermoid carcinoma.

This observation was followed by a long series of papers by Cherry and Glucksman in which female hooded Lister rats painted intravaginally with 1% DMBA in acetone were used as the model to study the role of the ovary, the effect of endocrine changes, the effect of castration with additional steroid or other hormones, and the effect of irradiation.[53] Their general conclusions were that the effect of these agents on cervical carcinogenesis by DMBA differed from their effects on normal target tissue of the cervicovaginal tract. For example, estrogens (which stimulated the growth of the cervicovaginal stroma, induced the multiplication of epithelial cells, and promoted keratinization) inhibited the development of sarcomas in a dose-dependent way in both intact and spayed females. Similarly, testosterone, cortisone, methylthiouracil, L-thyroxine, or repeated whole-body x rays (which do not stimulate stromal growth or epithelial keratinization) increased the rate of growth of tumors induced by DMBA. These apparently anomalous results may be complicated by the fact that DMBA itself has progesterone-mimetic effects.[84] They also noted that the histologic type of tumor that was induced was influenced to some extent by the various hormonal treatments.

These authors have shown similar results in mice treated with DMBA by the cervical painting method. Ovariectomy significantly increased the incidence of mucoepidermoid carcinoma of the cervix. Spayed females treated with progesterone had an increased adenocarcinomatous component, whereas stilbestrol gave only squamous cell carcinoma.[55]

Carcinogen paintings of the cervix and vagina often result in contamination of the vulva and this leads to marked hyperplasia, papillomas, and finally squamous carcinoma, all changes similar to those induced in normal skin with carcinogen painting. In mice it was shown that ovariectomy, which had little effect on cervical tumors induced by DMBA, increased the incidence of vulval tumors significantly.[56]

Induction of vulval tumors in rats painted with DMBA was not influenced by estrogen administration, ovariectomy,[54] or irradiation, but the incidence did increase with the dose of DMBA used.[20] In another experiment, castration promoted progression of vulval papillomas to carcinoma.[56]

Experiments have also been performed in mice with DMBA-impregnated knotted silk, with and without estrogen or androgen. Testosterone accelerated tumor appearance; ovariectomy lowered the incidence, as did estrogen treatment of intact females. The majority of tumors seen were squamous cell carcinoma; there were also a few cases of adenocarcinoma and myosarcoma, but no particular group had a preponderance of one kind of tumor.[124] Cytogenetic analysis of these tumors has been made.[80] It was found to vary considerably, in contrast with that of thymic lymphomas induced by DMBA.

CARBOWAX 1000 (POLYETHYLENE GLYCOL). In testing spermicidal contraceptives for possible carcinogenesis in mice, test substances were dissolved in Carbowax 1000 and introduced into the vagina twice a week using a syringe with a blunt needle. Eighteen months later, tumors of the cervix and vagina were seen in five out of 11 control animals, which received only the carbowax. All the tumors were carcinoma. DMBA added to the Carbowax resulted in nine tumors in 10 animals in a period of 12 months.[16]

N, N^1-DIMETHYL-*N*-NITROSOUREA. Administration of this chemical by subcutaneous injection once a week to young adult Syrian hamsters, after 18 injections, resulted in adenoacanthomas of the uterus in 86% of test animals.[69]

Virus

Viruslike particles have been seen in examination of the ultrastructure of cervical carcinomas induced in (C3H × A) mice by treatment with BP. These particles were indistinguishable from those described in mammary tumors of these strains. They were not seen in any of the normal tissues of the mice that were examined and it was speculated that the virus particles seen in the tumors might be a result, rather than a cause, of the carcinomatous process.[190]

HERPESVIRUS TYPE 2 (HSV-2). Experiments have been done in order to attempt to induce cervical cancers in animals with this virus. The animals were infected by applying the virus on cotton wool swabs to the cervix. It is reported that rabbits treated in this way die with paralysis and encephalitis.[169] BALB/c mice treated with hormones (estrogen, progesterone, or Enovid) and with HSV-2 intravaginally (twice at the beginning and again after 10 months) show characteristic cytologic changes of herpes infection in 40%. No significant difference was seen in the frequency of cancerous or precancerous lesions of the cervix or vagina between those receiving HSV-2 with hormone and those receiving hormone alone. However, in 19 animals on HSV-2 alone, two cancers and one precancerous lesion were seen. One of these cancers was transplanted with success.[135]

Treatment of various nonhuman primates has also been tried. Rhesus and squirrel monkeys could not be infected. Baboons could be infected but did not show lesions. Marmosets could be infected but soon died. However, *Cebus* monkeys (*albifrons* or *apella*) were susceptible to genital infection and survived. Twelve strains of HSV-2 were used, each on at least two monkeys, and 11 of the strains caused genital infection. Five strains produced tumor. In a total of 89 female *Cebus* monkeys exposed to HSV-2 infection, 50% developed lesions on the vulva, the cervix, and occasionally on the mouth. Nineteen males were exposed to the infected females and cross-infection by venereal infection was noted in two. One had penile lesions similar to those in humans.[112]

Assessment of the Animal Tumor Models for Cancer of the Uterus

On the whole, the administration of steroid hormones to adult female animals is not a very effective way of obtaining a specific type of uterine tumor. These hormones have a multitude of target organs and tissues, leading to many unwanted side effects that may kill the animal before tumors have had time to develop at the desired uterine site. As with ovarian tumors, species and genotypes are important factors in determining the outcome. The age at which experimental treatment begins is also of importance and greater specificity of action can sometimes be obtained by treatment at very early ages, even *in utero.*

Induction methods using carcinogens are generally to be preferred. Chemical carcinogens can be made to deliver a much more localized and continuous action on the target tissue when knotted threads impregnated with them are sewn into a particular part of the reproductive tract. When they (or oncogenic viruses) are injected directly into exposed fetectomy sites, their action is also localized and effective in inducing only the desired tumor type.

Although spontaneous tumors of the female genital tract (particularly of the cervix) are uncommon in most animal species, they can be induced with varying degrees of reliability in laboratory animals and virtually all types of tumors seen in the human female have been encountered in one species or another. In describing their induction methods I have tried to show that chemical factors (chemical carcinogens); physical factors (irridiation, intrauterine devices); and biologic factors, both intrinsic (genetic factors, age, hormones) and extrinsic (viruses), may all play their part in causing cancer of the female reproductive tract. None of them can be neglected in the search for etiologic factors in the human species.

LABORATORY ANIMALS AS HOSTS FOR HUMAN TUMORS

The experimentally minded gynecologic oncologist may be interested in the utilization of laboratory animals as hosts for human tumor transplants. This enables study of the hormone dependence of a tumor to be made or the tumor's susceptibility to inhibition by drugs to be examined.

One system that allows such transplants to be maintained is the hamster cheek pouch. Transplantation of human trophoblastic tumors to this immunologically privileged site has shown profound inhibition of tumor growth by methotrexate.[67]

Another system is the immune-suppressed mouse, either genetically determined as in the "nude" athymic mice or induced as a result of neonatal thymectomy. In a recent investigation of 19 human malignant tumors inoculated into male and female "nude" hosts, nine showed exclusive or preferential growth in one sex only, suggesting a hormonal influence on a wide variety of human tumors.[52]

It is hoped that further study along these lines can lead to more effective treatment of human malignant disease.

REFERENCES

1. Allen, E., and Gardner, W. U. Cancer of the cervix of the uterus in hybrid mice following long-continued administration of estrogen. *Cancer Res. 1*:359, 1941.

2. Alvizouri, M., and de Pita, V. R. Experimental carcinoma of the cervix. Hormonal influences. *Am. J. Obstet. Gynecol. 89*:940, 1964.

3. Baba, N., and von Haam, E. Experimental carcinoma of the endometrium. Adenocarcinoma in rabbits and squamous cell carcinoma in rats and mice. *Prog. Exp. Tumor Res. 9*:192, 1967.

4. Baba, N., and von Haam, E. Squamous cell carcinoma of the rat endometrium produced by insertion of strings coated with paraffin and polymer. *J. Natl. Cancer Inst. 47*:675, 1971.

5. Bacon, R. R. Tumors of the epididymis and of the uterus in hamsters treated with diethylstilbestrol and testosterone propionate. *Cancer Res. 12*:246, 1952.

6. Bali, T., and Furth, J. Morphological and biological characteristics of X-ray induced transplantable ovarian tumors. *Cancer Res. 9*:449, 1949.

7. Barbieri, G., Olivi, M., and Sacco, O. Lesioni microscopiche nel' uteri di topi (BALB/C_f, C3H/CB/Se substrain) trattati con benzoato di estradiolo. *Lav. Ist. Anat. Istol. Patol. Perugia 18*:165, 1958.

8. Biancifiori, C., Bonser, G. M., and Caschera, F. Ovarian and mammary tumours in intact C3Hb virgin mice following a limited dose of four carcinogenic chemicals. *Br. J. Cancer 15*:270, 1961.

9. Bielschowsky, F., and Hall, W. H. Carcinogenesis in parabiotic rats. Tumours of the ovary induced by acetylaminofluorene in intact females joined to gonadectomised littermates and the reaction of their pituitaries to endogenous oestrogens. *Br. J. Cancer 5*:331, 1951.

10. Bielschowsy, M., and D'Ath, E. F. Spontaneous granulosa cell tumours of mice of strain NZC-Bi, NZO-Bi, NZY-Bi and NZB-Bi. *Pathology 5*:303, 1973.

11. Biskind, G. R., Bernstein, D. E., and Gospe, S. M. The effect of

exogenous gonadotrophins on the development of experimental ovarian tumors in rats. *Cancer Res. 13*:216, 1953.

12. Biskind, G. R., and Biskind, M. S. Experimental ovarian tumors in rats. *Am. J. Clin. Pathol. 19*:501, 1949.

13. Biskind, G. R., Kordan, B., and Biskind, M. S. Ovary transplanted to spleen in rats: The effect of unilateral castration, pregnancy and subsequent castration. *Cancer Res. 10*:309, 1950.

14. Bonser, G. M., and Jull, J. W. Tumours of the Ovary. Personal communication, 1974.

15. Bonser, G. M., and Robson, J. M. The induction of tumours following the direct implantation of 20-methylcholanthrene in the uterus of mice. *Br. J. Cancer 4*:196, 1950.

16. Boyland, E., Charles, R. T., and Gowing, N. F. C. The induction of tumours in mice by intravaginal application of chemical compounds. *Br. J. Cancer 15*:252, 1961.

17. Bruzzone, S., and Lipschutz, A. Endometrial adenocarcinoma and extragenital tumours in guinea-pigs with 'ovarian fragmentation'. *Br. J. Cancer 8*:613, 1954.

18. Bullock, F. D., and Curtis, M. R. Spontaneous tumors of the rat. *J. Cancer Res. 14*:1, 1930.

19. Carter, R. L. Pathology of ovarian neoplasms in rats and mice. *Eur. J. Cancer 3*:537, 1968.

20. Cherry, C. P., and Glucksman, A. The effect of endocrine changes, of irradiation and of additional treatment of the skin on the induction of tumours in the female genital tract of rats by chemical carcinogens. *Br. J. Cancer 14*:489, 1960.

21. Christov, K., and Raichev, R. Proliferative and neoplastic changes in the ovaries of hamsters treated with 131-iodine and methylthiouracil. *Neoplasma 20*:511, 1973.

22. Corfman, P. A., and Richart, R. M. Induction in rats of uterine epidermoid carcinomas by plastic and stainless steel intrauterine devices. *Am. J. Obstet. Gynecol. 98*:987, 1967.

23. Cotchin, E. Spontaneous uterine cancer in animals. *Br. J. Cancer 18*:209, 1964.

24. Damjanov, I., and Solter, D. Host related factors determine outgrowth of terato-carcinomas from mouse egg-cylinders. *Z. Krebsforsch. 81*:63, 1974.

25. Davies, J., and Kusama, H. Developmental aspects of the human cervix. *Ann. N.Y. Acad. Sci. 97*:534, 1962.

26. Dawson, P. J., Brooks, R. E., and Fieldsteel, A. H. Unusual occurrence of endometrial sarcomas in hybrid mice. *J. Natl. Cancer Inst. 52*:207, 1974.

27. Deringer, M. K. Occurrence of tumors, particularly mammary tumors, in agent-free strain C3HeB mice. *J. Natl. Cancer Inst. 22*:995, 1959.

28. Deringer, M. K., Lorenz, E., and Uphoff, D. E. Fertility and tumor development in (C57L $\times$ A)F_1 hybrid mice receiving X radiation to ovaries only, to whole body, and to whole body with ovaries shielded. *J. Natl. Cancer Inst. 15*:931, 1954.

29. Dickie, M. M. The use of F_1 hybrid and backcross generations to reveal new and/or uncommon tumour types. *J. Natl. Cancer Inst. 15*:791, 1954.

30. Dunn, T. B. The importance of differences in morphology in inbred strains. *J. Natl. Cancer. Inst. 15*:573, 1954.

31. Dunn, T. B. Cancer of the uterine cervix in mice fed a liquid diet containing anti-fertility drug. *J. Natl. Cancer Inst. 43*:671, 1969.

32. Dunn, T. B., and Green, A. W. Cysts of the epididymis, cancer of the cervix, granular cell myoblastoma, and other lesions after estrogen injection in newborn mice. *J. Natl. Cancer Inst. 31*:425, 1963.

33. Fawcett, D. W. Bilateral ovarian teratomas in a mouse. *Cancer Res. 10*:705, 1950.

34. Fekete, E., and Ferrigno, M. A. Studies on a transplantable teratoma of the mouse. *Cancer Res. 12*:438, 1952.

35. Fels, E. Effet de la ligature tubaire sur la fonction ovarienne chez le rat. *C. R. Soc. Biol. 148*:1666, 1954.

36. Fels, E. Aspectos morfológicos y funcionales de los tumores experimentales del ovario. *Rev. Arg. Endocrinol. Metab. 2*:1, 1956.

37. Fishman, M., Shear, M. J., Friedman, H. F., and Stewart, H. L. Studies in carcinogenesis. XVII. Local effect of repeated application of 3,4-Benzpyrene and of human smegma to the vagina and cervix of mice. *J. Natl. Cancer Inst. 2*:361, 1941–2.

38. Flux, J. E. C. Incidence of ovarian tumors in hares in New Zealand. *J. Wildlife Mgmnt. 29*:622, 1965.

39. Forsber, J. G. Estrogen, vaginal cancer and vaginal development. *Am. J. Obstet. Gynecol. 113*:83, 1972.

40. Forsberg, J. C., and Breitstein, L. S. Carcinogenesis with 3-methylcholanthrene in uterine cervix of mice treated neonatally with estrogen. *J. Natl. Cancer Inst. 49*:155, 1972.

41. Furth, J., and Boon, M. C. Induction of ovarian tumors in mice by X-rays. *Cancer Res. 7*:241, 1947.

42. Furth, J., and Furth, O. B. Neoplastic diseases produced in mice by general irradiation with X-rays. *Am. J. Cancer 28*:54, 1936.

43. Furth, J., and Sobel, H. Neoplastic transformations of granulosa cells in grafts of normal ovaries into spleens of gonadectomised mice. *J. Natl. Cancer Inst. 8*:7, 1947.

44. Furth, J., and Sobel, H. Transplantable luteoma in mice and associated secondary changes. *Cancer Res. 7*:246, 1947.

45. Gardner, W. U. Studies on steroid hormones in experimental carcinogenesis. *Rec. Prog. Horm. Res. 1*:217, 1947.

46. Gardner, W. U. Further studies on experimental ovarian tumorigenesis. *Proc. Am. Assoc. Cancer Res. 2*:300, 1958.

47. Gardner, W. U. Carcinoma of the uterine cervix and upper vagina: Induction under experimental conditions in mice. *Ann. N.Y. Acad. Sci. 75*:543, 1959.

48. Gardner, W. U. Tumorigenesis in transplanted irradiated and nonirradiated ovaries. *J. Natl. Cancer Inst. 26*:829, 1961.

49. Gardner, W. U., Allan, E., and Strong, L. C. Atypical uterine and vaginal changes in mice receiving large doses of estrogenic hormone. *Anat. Rec. 64*:17, Suppl. 3 (Abstract), 1936.

50. Gardner, W. U., and Ferrigno, M. Unusual neoplastic lesions of the uterine horns of estrogen-treated mice. *J. Natl. Cancer Inst. 17*:601, 1956.

51. Gardner, W. U., and Pan, S. C. Malignant tumors of the uterus and vagina in untreated mice of the PM stock. *Cancer Res. 8*:241, 1948.

52. Giovanella, B. C., and Stehlin, J. S. Influence of the host's sex on the growth of human tumors heterotransplanted in "nude" thymusless mice. *Am. Assoc. Cancer Res., 15*, Abstract 92, 1974.

53. Glucksman, A. Some effects of steroid hormones on carcinogenesis in rats: Effects of oestrogens on the induction of tumours in the cervico-vaginal tract and in the salivary glands, in Williams, D. C., and Briggs, M. C., eds.: *Some Implications of Steroid Hormones in Cancer*. London, Heinemann Medical Books, 1971, pp. 70–78.

54. Glucksman, A., and Cherry, C. P. The role of the ovary in the induction of tumours by the local application of 9,10-dimethyl-1,2-benzanthracene to the genital tract of rats. *Br. J. Cancer 12*:32, 1958.

55. Glucksman, A., and Cherry, C. P. The effect of castration and of additional hormonal treatments on the induction of cervical and vulval tumours in mice. *Br. J. Cancer 16*:634, 1962.

56. Glucksman, A., and Cherry, C. P. The effect of increased numbers of carcinogenic treatments on the induction of cervico-vaginal and vulval tumours in intact and castrate rats. *Br. J. Cancer 24*:333, 1970.

57. Gorski, R. A., and Wagner, J. W. Gonadal activity and sexual differentiation of the hypothalamus. *Endocrinology 76*:226, 1965.

58. Graham, C. E. Cyclic changes in the squamo-columnar junction of the mouse cervix uteri. *Anat. Rec. 155*:251, 1966.

59. Graham, C. E. Relationship of carcinogenesis and epidermization during 20-methylcholanthrene treatment of the mouse uterine cervix. *Am. J. Obstet. Gynecol. 103*:1084, 1969.

60. Greene, H. S. N. Adenocarcinoma of the uterine fundus in the rabbit. *Ann. N.Y. Acad. Sci. 75*:535, 1959.

61. Greenwood, A. W. Controlled environments and cancer incidence in the domestic fowl, in Shives, A. A., ed.: *Racial and Geographical Factors in Tumour Incidence. Medical Monograph 2.* Edinburgh, University Press, 1967, pp. 241–249.

62. Guthrie, M. J. Tumorigenesis in intrasplenic ovaries in mice. *Cancer, N.Y. 10*:190, 1957.

63. Hafez, E. S. E. The comparative anatomy of the mammalian cervix in Blandau, R. J., and Moghissi, K., eds.: *The Biology of the Cervix.* Chicago, Chicago University Press, 1973, Ch. 3.

64. Hale, H. B., and Weichert, C. K. Ovarian tumors in adult rats following prepuberal administration of estrogens. *Proc. Soc. Exp. Biol. Med. 55*:201, 1944.

65. Hamilton, C. E. The cervix uteri of the rat. *Anat. Rec. 97*:47, 1947.

66. Herbst, A. L., Ulfelder, H., and Poskanzer, D. C. Adenocarcinoma of the vagina—association of maternal stilboestrol therapy with the tumor appearance in young women. *N. Engl. J. Med. 284*:878, 1971.

67. Hertz, R. Biological aspects of gestational neoplasms derived from trophoblast. *Ann. N.Y. Acad. Sci. 172*:279, 1971.

68. Hilfrich, J. A new model for inducing malignant ovarian tumours in rats. *Br. J. Cancer 28*:46, 1973.

69. Hiraki, S. Carcinogenic effect of *N,N'*-dimethylnitrosourea on Syrian hamsters. *Gann 62*:321, 1971.

70. Homburger, F. Chemical carcinogenesis in Syrian hamsters. *Prog. Exp. Tumor Res. 16*:152, 1972.

71. Hori, C. G., Warren, S., Patterson, W. B., and Chute, R. N. Gamma ray induction of malignant tumors in rats. *Am. J. Pathol. 65*:279, 1971.

72. Horning, E. S. Carcinogenic action of androgens. *Br. J. Cancer 64*:414, 1958.

73. Howell, J. S., Marchant, J., and Orr, J. W. The induction of ovarian tumors in mice with 9:10-dimethyl-1;2-benzanthracene. *Br. J. Cancer 8*:635, 1954.

74. Huggins, C. B., and Sugiyama, T. Production and prevention of two distinctive kinds of destruction of the adrenal cortex. *Nature (London) 206*:1310, 1965.

75. Hummel, K. P. Induced ovarian tumors. *J. Natl. Cancer Inst. 15*:711, 1954.

76. Iglesias, R. Newer concepts in pathogenesis. Secondary endocrine and mammary malignancies as main signs of hormonal syndromes produced by endocrine tumors. *Ann. N.Y. Acad. Sci. 230*:500, 1974.

77. Iglesias, R., Mardones, E., and Lipschutz, A. Evolution of luteoma in intrasplenic ovarian grafts in the guinea-pig. *Br. J. Cancer 7*:214, 1953.

78. Iijima, H., Nasu, K., and Taki, I. Comparative study of carcinogenesis in squamous columnar epithelium of mouse uterus by string method of producing cervical carcinoma. *Am. J. Obstet. Gynecol. 89*:946, 1964.

79. Jabara, A. G. Induction of canine ovarian tumours by diethylstilboestrol and progesterone. *Aust. J. Exp. Biol. Med. Sci. 40*:139, 1962.

80. Joneja, M. J., and Coulson, D. B. Histopathology and cytogenetics of tumors induced by the application of 7,12-dimethylbenz[*a*]anthracene (DMBA) in mouse cervix. *Eur. J. Cancer 9*:367, 1973.

81. Jones, D. C., and Witschi, E. Endocrinology of ovarian tumor formation in parabiotic rats. *Cancer Res. 21*:783, 1961.

82. Jones, E. C., and Krohn, P. L. Influence of the anterior pituitary on the ageing process in the ovary. *Nature (London) 183*:1155, 1959.

83. Jones, E. C., and Krohn, P. L. The relationships between age, numbers of oocytes and fertility in virgin and multiparous mice. *J. Endocrinol. 21*:469, 1961.

84. Jull, J. W. Hormones as promoting agents in mammary carcinogenesis. *Acta Un. Int. Cancer (Louvain) 12*:653, 1956.

85. Jull, J. W. Mechanism of induction of ovarian tumors in the mouse by 7,12-dimethylbenz[*a*]anthracene. VI Effect of normal ovarian tissue on tumor development. *J. Natl. Cancer Inst. 42*:967, 1969.

86. Jull, J. W. Ovarian tumorigenesis. *Methods Cancer Res. 7*:131, 1973.

87. Jull, J. W., Hawryluk, A., and Russell, A. Mechanism of induction of ovarian tumors in the mouse by 7,12-dimethylbenz[*a*]anthracene. III Tumor induction in organ culture. *J. Natl. Cancer Inst. 40*:687, 1968.

88. Jull, J. W., and Jellink, P. H. Mechanism of induction of ovarian tumors in the mouse by 7,12-dimethylbenz[*a*]anthracene. IV Uptake and retention of C^{14}—DMBA by mouse and rat tissues. *J. Natl. Cancer Inst. 40*:707, 1968.

89. Jull, J. W., and Russell, A. Mechanism of induction of ovarian tumors in the mouse by 7,12-dimethylbenz[*a*]anthracene. VII Relative activities of parent hydrocarbon and some of its metabolites. *J. Natl. Cancer Inst. 44*:841, 1970.

90. Jurow, H. N. Cyclic variations in the cervix of the guinea-pig. *Am. J. Obstet. Gynecol. 45*:762, 1943.

91. Kaminetzky, H. A. Methylcholanthrene-induced cervical dysplasia and the sex steroids. *Obstet. Gynecol. 27*:489, 1966.

92. Kimura, T., and Nandi, S. Nature of induced persistent vaginal cornification in mice. IV Changes in the vaginal epithelium of old mice treated neonatally with estradiol or testosterone. *J. Natl. Cancer Inst. 39*:75, 1967.

93. Kirkman, H. Hormone-related tumors in Syrian hamsters. *Prog. Exp. Tumor Res. 16*:201, 1972.

94. Kirkman, H., and Algard, F. T. Characteristics of an androgen/estrogen induced uterine smooth muscle tumor of the Syrian hamster. *Cancer Res. 30*:794, 1970.

95. Koprowska, I., Bogacz, J., Pentikas, C., and Stypulkowski, W. Induced cervical carcinoma of the mouse. A quantitative cytological method for evaluation of the neoplastic process. *Cancer Res. 18*:1186, 1958.

96. Krarup, T. 9:10-dimethyl-1:2-benzanthracene induced ovarian tumours in mice. *Acta Pathol. Microbiol. Scand. 70*:241, 1967.

97. Krarup, T. Oocyte destruction and ovarian tumorigenesis

after direct application of a chemical carcinogen (9:10-dimethyl-1:2-benzanthracene) to the mouse ovary. *Intl. J. Cancer 4*:61, 1969.

98. Krarup, T., and Loft, H. Presence of DMBA-^{3}H in the mouse ovary and its relation to ovarian tumour induction. *Acta Pathol. Microbiol. Scand. A 79*:139, 1971.

99. Kullander, S. On tumor formation in gonadal and hypophyseal transplants into the anterior eye chambers of gonadectomised rats. *Cancer Res. 20*:1079, 1960.

100. Kushima, K., Noda, K., and Makita, M. Experimental production of chorionic tumor in rabbits. *Tohuko J. Med. 91*:209, 1967.

101. Kuwahara, I. Experimental induction of ovarian tumors in mice treated with single administration of 7,12-dimethylbenz[*a*]anthracene, and its pathological observation. *Gann 58*:253, 1967.

102. Lee, S., Condon, J. K., Chandler, J. G., Koopmans, H., Ehara, Y., Yen, S. S., and Orloff, M. J. The effect of Eck fistula upon intrasplenic ovarian neoplasm formation. *Surg. Forum 23*:110, 1972.

103. Li, M. H., and Gardner, W. U. Further studies on the pathogenesis of ovarian tumors in mice. *Cancer Res. 9*:35, 1949.

104. Lick, L., Kirschbaum, A., and Mixer, H. Mechanism of induction of ovarian tumors by X-rays. *Cancer Res. 9*:532, 1949.

105. Lipschutz, A. *Steroid Homeostasis. Hypophysis and Tumorigenesis.* Cambridge, Heffer and Sons, 1957.

106. Lipschutz, A., Iglesias, R., Panasevich, V. I., and Salinas, S. Granulosa-cell tumours induced in mice by progesterone. *Br. J. Cancer 21*:144, 1967.

107. Lipschutz, A., Iglesias, R., Panasevich, V. I., and Salinas, S. Pathological changes induced in the uterus of mice with the prolonged administration of progesterone and 19-nor-contraceptives. *Br. J. Cancer 21*:160, 1967.

108. Lipschutz, A., Iglesias, R., Panasevich, V. I., and Socorro, S. Ovarian tumours and other ovarian changes induced in mice by two 19-nor-contraceptives. *Br. J. Cancer 21*:153, 1967.

109. Lipschutz, A., Iglesias, R., Salinas, S., and Panasevich, V. I. Experimental conditions under which contraceptive steroids may become toxic. *Nature (London) 212*:686, 1966.

110. Lipschutz, A., and Vargas, L. Structure and origin of uterine and extragenital fibroids induced experimentally in the guinea-pig by prolonged administration of estrogens. *Cancer Res. 1*:236, 1941.

111. Loeb, L., Burns, E. L., Suntzeff, V., and Moskop, M. Carcinoma-like proliferations in vagina, cervix and uterus of mouse treated with estrogens. *Proc. Soc. Exp. Biol. Med. 35*:320, 1936.

112. London, W. T., Nahmias, A. J., Naib, Z. M., Fucillo, D. A., Ellenberg, J. H., and Sever, J. L. A nonhuman primate model for the study of the cervical oncogenic potential of *Herpes simplex* virus type 2. *Cancer Res. 34*:1118, 1974.

113. Lorenz, E. Some biologic effects of long continued radiation. *Am. J. Roentgenol Radium Ther. Nucl. Med. 63*:176, 1950.

114. Manocha, S. L., and Graham, C. E. Histochemistry of mouse cervical epithelium during chemical carcinogenesis. *Histochem. J. 2*:357, 1970.

115. Marchant, J. Influence of the strain of ovarian grafts on the induction of breast and ovarian tumours in F_1 (C57B1 × IF) hybrid mice by 9:10-dimethyl-1:2-benzanthracene. *Br. J. Cancer 13*:306, 1959.

116. Marchant, J. Changes in the ovaries of mice treated with dimethylbenzanthracene and observations on the subsequent development of tumours in ovaries and breasts. *Br. J. Cancer 13*:652, 1959.

117. Marchant, J. The development of ovarian tumours in ovaries grafted from mice pretreated with dimethylbenzanthracene. Inhibition by the presence of normal ovarian tissue. Br. J. Cancer *14*:514, 1960.

118. Marchant, J. The effect of hypophysectomy on the development of ovarian tumours in mice treated with dimethylbenzanthracene. *Br. J. Cancer 15*:821, 1961.

119. Marchant, J. Personal observation, 1960.

120. Marchant, J., Orr, J. W., and Woodhouse, D. L. Induction of ovarian tumors with 9:10-dimethyl-1:2-benzanthracene. *Nature (London) 173*:307, 1954.

121. Mardones, E., Iglesias, R., and Lipschutz, A. Granulosa cell tumours in intrasplenic ovarian grafts, with intrahepatic metastases, in guinea-pigs at five years after grafting. *Br. J. Cancer 9*:409, 1955.

122. McClure, H. M., and Graham, C. E. Malignant uterine mesotheliomas in squirrel monkeys following diethylstilboestrol administration. *Lab. Anim. Sci. 23*:493, 1973.

123. Meier, H., Myers, D. D., Fox, R. R., and Laird, C. W. Occurrence, pathological features, and propagation of gonadal teratomas in inbred mice and rabbits. *Cancer Res. 30*:30, 1970.

124. Meisels, A. Effect of sex hormones on the carcinogenic action of dimethylbenzanthracene on the uterus of intact and castrated mice. *Cancer Res. 26*:757, 1966.

125. Meissner, W. A., Sommers, S. C., and Sherman, G. Endometrial hyperplasia, endometrial carcinoma, and endometriosis produced experimentally by estrogen. *Cancer, N.Y. 10*:500, 1957.

126. Miller, O. J., and Gardner, W. U. The role of thyroid function and food intake in experimental ovarian tumorigenesis in mice. *Cancer Res. 14*:220, 1954.

127. Mody, J. K. The action of four carcinogenic hydrocarbons on the ovaries of IF mice and the histogenesis of induced tumours. *Br. J. Cancer 14*:256, 1960.

128. Moon, H. D., Simpson, M. E., Li, C. H., and Evans, H. M. Neoplasms in rats and mice treated with pituitary growth hormone. III Reproductive organs. *Cancer Res. 10*:549, 1950.

129. Mossman, H. W. The embryology of the cervix. *In* Blandau, R. J., and Moghissi, K. eds.: *The Biology of the Cervix*. Chicago, Chicago University Press, 1973, Ch. 2.

130. Mossman, H. W., and Duke, K. L. *Comparative Morphology of the Mammalian* Ovary. Madison University of Wisconsin Press, 1973.

131. Mühlbock, O. Hormonale ovariumtumoren na Röntgenbestraling. *Ned. Tijdsch. v. Geneesk., 95*:915, 1951.

132. Mühlbock, O. Ovarian tumours in mice in parabiotic union. *Acta Endocrinol.* Copenhagen. 12:105, 1953.

133. Mühlbock, O. On the genesis of ovarian tumours. Experiments with mice in parabiotic union. *Acta Un. Int. Cancr (Louvain) 10*:141, 1954.

134. Mühlbock, O., van Nie, R., and Bosch, L. The production of oestrogenic hormones by granulosa cell tumours in mice, in *Hormone Production in Endocrine Tumours,* Ciba Found. Colloq. Endocrinol., 1958, Vol. 12, p. 78.

135. Muñoz, N. Effect of Herpesvirus Type 2 and hormonal imbalance on the uterine cervix of the mouse. *Cancer Res. 33*:1504, 1973.

136. Murphy, E. D. Carcinogenesis of the uterine cervix in mice: Effect of diethylstilbestrol after limited application of 3-methylcholanthrene. *J. Natl. Cancer Inst. 27*:611, 1961.

137. Murphy, E. D. Characteristic tumors, in Green, E. L., ed:

Jackson Laboratory. *Biology of the Laboratory Mouse,* 2nd ed. New York, McGraw Hill, 1966, Ch. 27.

138. Murphy, E. D. Carcinogenesis of the uterine cervix in mice: Effect of castration after limited application of 3-methylcholanthrene. *J. Natl. Cancer Inst. 41:*1111, 1968.

139. Murphy, E. D. Hyperplastic and early neoplastic changes in the ovaries of mice after genic deletion of germ cells. *J. Natl. Cancer Inst. 48:*1283, 1972.

140. Murphy, E. D., and Beamer, W. G. Plasma gonadotropin levels during early stages of ovarian tumorigenesis in mice of the W^x/W^v genotype. *Cancer Res. 33:*721, 1973.

141. Nairn, R. C., Wallace, A. C., and Guli, E. P. Intestinal antigenicity of ovarian mucinous cystadenomas. *Br. J. Cancer 25:*276, 1971.

142. Nelson, L. W., Kelly, W. A., and Weikel, J. H. Mesovarial leiomyomas in rats in a chronic toxicity study of mesuprine hydrochloride. *Toxicol. Appl. Pharmacol. 23:*731, 1972.

143. Nelson, W. O. Atypical uterine growths produced by prolonged administration of estrogenic hormones. *Endocrinology 24:*50, 1939.

144. Nishizuka, Y., and Sakakura, T. Ovarian dysgenesis induced by neonatal thymectomy in the mouse. *Endocrinology 89:*886, 1971.

145. Nishizuka, Y., and Sakakura, T. Effect of combined removal of thymus and pituitary on post-natal ovarian follicular development in the mouse. *Endocrinology 89:*902, 1971.

146. Nishizuka, Y., Tanaka, Y., Sakakura, T., and Kojma, A. Frequent development of ovarian tumors from dysgenetic ovaries of neonatally thymectomised mice. *Gann 63:*139, 1972.

147. Nomura, T. Carcinogenesis by urethane via mother's milk and its enhancement of transplacental carcinogenesis in mice. *Cancer Res. 33:*1677, 1973.

148. Nomura, T., Okamoto, E., and Manabe, H. Ovarian teratoma found in an offspring of mothers (ICR-JCL mice) treated with urethane. *Med. J. Osaka Univ. 23:*121, 1972.

149. Oakberg, E. F. Effect of 25R of X-rays at 10 days of age on oocyte numbers and fertility of female mice, in Lindop, D. J., and Sacher, G. A., eds.: *Radiation and Ageing.* London, Taylor and Francis, 1966, pp. 293–306.

150. Pan, S. C., and Gardner, W. U. Induction of malignant tumors by methylcholanthrene in transplanted uterine cornua and cervixes of mice. *Cancer Res. 8:*613, 1948.

151. Pantelouris, E. M. Athymic development in the mouse. *Differentiation 1:*437, 1973.

152. Peckham, B. M., and Greene, R. R. Experimentally produced granulosa-cell tumors in rabbits. *Cancer Res. 12:*654, 1952.

153. Perry, I. H., and Ginzton, L. L. The development of tumors in female mice treated with 1;2;5;6-dibenzanthracene and theelin. *Am. J. Cancer 29:*680, 1937.

154. Peters, H. Effects of radiation in early life on the morphology and reproductive function of the mouse ovary. *Adv. Reprod. Physiol. 4:*149, 1969.

155. Pfeiffer, C. A. Sexual differences of the hypophysis and their determination by the gonads. *Am. J. Anat. 58:*195, 1936.

156. Pfeiffer, C. A. Development of leiomyomas in female rats with an endocrine imbalance. *Cancer Res. 9:*277, 1949.

157. Pfeiffer, C. A. Adenocarcinoma in the uterus of an endocrine imbalance female rat. *Cancer Res. 9:*347, 1949.

158. Pierson, H. Experimental production of uterine enlargement with cancer through ovarian hormone. *Ztschr. Krebsforsch. 41:*103, 1934.

159. Reagen, J. W., Wentz, B. W., and Hachico, N. Induced cancer of the mouse. *Arch. Pathol. 6:*451, 1955.

160. Reboud, S., and Pageant, G. Co-carcinogenic effect of progesterone on 20-methylcholanthrene-induced cervical carcinoma in mice. *Nature (London) 241:*398, 1973.

161. Reuber, M. D. Endometrial sarcomas of the uterus and carcinosarcoma of the submaxillary salivary gland in castrated A × C strain female rats receiving *N,N′*-fluorenyldiacetamide and norethandrolone. *J. Natl. Cancer Inst. 25:*1141, 1960.

162. Roberts, D. C. Transplanted tumours of the Golden hamster (*Mesocricetus auratus*) used in research 1964–1970. *Prog. Exp. Tumor. Res. 16:*558, 1972.

163. Rubio, C. A., and Lagelöf, B. Studies on the histogenesis of experimentally induced cervical carcinoma. *Acta Pathol. Microbiol. Scand. A 82:*153, 1974.

164. Rubio, C. A., and Lagelöf, B. Autoradiographic studies of experimentally induced atypias in the cervical epithelium of mice. *Acta Pathol. Microbiol. Scand. A 82:*475, 1974.

165. Russell, E. S., and Fekete, E. Analysis of W-series pleiotropism in the mouse: Effect of W^vW^v substitution on definitive germ cells and on ovarian tumorigenesis. *J. Natl. Cancer Inst. 21:*365, 1958.

166. Scarpelli, D. G., and von Haam, E. Experimental carcinoma of the uterine cervix in the mouse. *Am. J. Pathol. 33:*1059, 1957.

167. Sekiya, S., Takamizawa, H., Wang, F., Takane, T., and Kuwata, T. In vivo and in vitro studies on uterine adenocarcinoma of the rat induced by 7,12-dimethylbenz[*a*]anthracene. *Am. J. Obstet. Gynecol. 113:*691, 1972.

168. Sekiya, S., Yam, A., and Takamizawa, H. Enhancement of tumor growth and metastases by medroxyprogesterone acetate in transplanted uterine adenocarcinoma cells of the rat. *J. Natl. Cancer Inst. 52:*297, 1974.

169. Sever, J. L. Herpes virus and cervical cancer studies in experimental animals. *Cancer Res. 33:*1509, 1973.

170. Shen, C. N. Experimental induction of placental tumor in the guinea pig. *Nagoya Med. J. 17:*33, 1971.

171. Shintani, S., Glass, L. E., and Page, E. W. Studies of induced malignant tumors of placental and uterine origin in the rat. II Induced tumors and pathogenesis. *Am. J. Obstet. Gynecol. 95:*550, 1966.

172. Shisa, H., and Nishizuka, Y. Unilateral development of ovarian tumour in thymectomized Swiss mice following a single injection of 7,12-dimethylbenz[*a*]anthracene at neonatal stage. *Br. J. Cancer 22:*70, 1968.

173. Singh, K. B. Induction of polycystic ovarian disease in rats by continuous light. I. The reproductive cycle, organ weights and histology of the ovaries. *Am. J. Obstet. Gynecol. 103:*1078, 1969.

174. Slye, M., Holmes, M. F., and Wells, H. G. Primary spontaneous tumors of the ovary in mice. *J. Cancer Res. 5:*205, 1920.

175. Sobis, H., and Vandeputte, M. Development of teratomas from displaced visceral yolk sac. *Intl. J. Cancer 13:*444, 1974.

176. Sommers, S. C., and Meissner. W. A. Host relationship in experimental endometrial carcinoma. *Cancer, N.Y. 10:*510, 1957.

177. Staats, J. Standardised nomenclature for inbred strains of mice. Third listing. *Cancer Res. 24:*147, 1964.

178. Stein-Werblowsky, R. Induction of cancer of the cervix in relation to the oestrus cycle. *Br. J. Cancer 14:*300, 1960.

179. Stevens, L. C. Experimental production of testicular teratomas in mice. *Proc. Natl. Acad. Sci. USA 52:*654, 1964.

180. Stevens, L. C., and Varnum, D. S. The development of teratomas from parthenogenetically activated ovarian mouse eggs. *Dev. Biol. 37:*369, 1974.

181. Strong, L. C., Gardner, W. U., and Hill, R. T. Production of estrogenic hormone by a transplantable ovarian carcinoma. *Endocrinology 21*:268, 1937.

182. Suntzeff, V., Burns, E. L., Moskop, M., and Loeb, L. On proliferative changes taking place in epithelium of vagina and cervix of mice with advancing age and under influence of experimentally administered estrogenic hormones. *Am. J. Cancer 32*:256, 1938.

183. Symeonides, A. Tumors induced by 2-acetylaminofluorene in virgin and breeding females of five strains of rats and in their offspring. *J. Natl. Cancer Inst. 15*:539, 1954.

184. Symeonides, A., and Mori-Chavez, P. A transplantable ovarian papillary adenocarcinoma of the rat with ascites implants in the ovary. *J. Natl. Cancer Inst. 13*:409, 1952.

185. Takamizawa, H., and Wong, K. Effect of anticancer drugs on uterine carcinogenesis. *Obstet. Gynecol. 41*:701, 1973.

186. Takasugi, N. Carcinogenesis by vaginal transplants from ovariectomized, neonatally-estrogenized mice into ovariectomized normal host. *Gann 63*:73, 1972.

187. Taki, I., and Iijima, H. A new method of producing endometrial cancer in mice. *Am. J. Obstet. Gynecol. 87*:926, 1963.

188. Taki, I., Iijima, H., Doi, T., Uetsuki, Y., and Masahiko, M. Histochemistry of hydrolytic and oxydative enzymes in the human and experimentally induced adenocarcinoma of the endometrium. *Am. J. Obstet. Gynecol. 94*:86, 1966.

189. Thiery, M. Ovarian teratoma in the mouse. *Br. J. Cancer 17*:231, 1936.

190. Thiery, M., De Groodt, M., De Rom, F., Sebryns, M., and Lagasse, A. Viruslike particles in chemically-induced carcinoma of the uterine cervix. *Nature (London) 183*:694, 1959.

191. Thiery, M., and Willighagen, R. G. J. Enzyme histochemistry of induced and transplanted squamous cell carcinoma of the uterine cervix. *Br. J. Cancer 18*:582, 1964.

192. Uematsu, K., and Huggins, C. B. Induction of leukaemia and ovarian tumors in mice by pulse-doses of aromatic hydrocarbons. *Mol. Pharmacol. 4*:427, 1968.

193. Vandeputte, M., Sobis, H., Billiau, A., van de Maele, B., and Leyten R. *In utero* tumor induction by murine sarcoma virus (Maloney) in the rat. I. Biological characteristics. *Intl. J. Cancer 11*:536, 1973.

194. van Nie, R., Benedetti, E. L., and Mühlbock, O. A carcinogenic action of testosterone, provoking uterine tumours in mice. *Nature (London) 192*:1303, 1961.

195. van Nie, R., Smit, G. M. J., and Mühlbock, O. The induction of uterine tumours in mice treated with testosterone. *Acta Un. Int. Cancer 18*:194, 1962.

196. Vellios, F., and Griffin, J. The pathogenesis of dimethylbenzanthracene-induced carcinoma of the cervix in rats. *Cancer Res. 17*:364, 1955.

197. Vesselinovich, S. D., Mihailovich, N., Rao, K. V., and Itze, L. Perinatal carcinogenesis by urethane. *Cancer Res. 31*:2143, 1971.

198. Vink, H. H. Ovarian teratomas in guinea pigs: A report of ten cases. *J. Pathol. 102*:180, 1970.

199. von Haam, E., and Scarpielli, D. G. Experimental carcinoma of the cervix: A comparative cytologic and histologic study. *Cancer Res. 15*:449, 1955.

200. Willis, R. A. Ovarian teratomas in guinea pigs. *J. Pathol. Bacteriol. 84*:237, 1962.

201. Yong, H. Y., and Campbell, J. S. Evolution of dysplasia of the uterine cervix and vagina induced by low dosages of carcinogen in mice. *Obstet. Gynecol. 26*:91, 1965.

E. Cotchin,
D.Sc., F.R.C.V.S., F.R.C. Path.

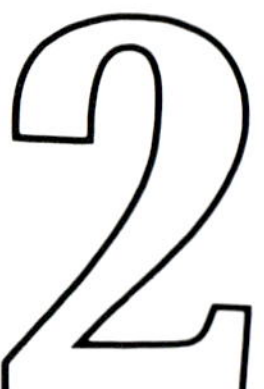

Spontaneous Tumors of the Uterus and Ovaries in Animals

General Introduction

In this chapter, a survey is made of the spontaneous tumors of the uterus and ovaries in animals. The bulk of information is about such tumors in domesticated animals, but some reference is also made to tumors in laboratory animals, wild animals, and animals in zoos. This is not a fully comprehensive bibliographic review but highlights the features of these tumors that appear to me, a veterinary pathologist, to be of most interest.

A note of caution may be sounded for those who are approaching the subject of spontaneous tumors in animals for the first time. Information about such tumors is inferior in quantity, and sometimes in quality, to that about tumors in humans.[40] Most of the reported studies of material from domesticated animals have been based on the histopathologic examination of biopsy or autopsy specimens in laboratories servicing the clinics in veterinary schools or examining material submitted by practitioners, although information has also been obtained from studies of abattoir material. As regards material from clinics and private practices, a considerable element of selection bias arises because the affected animal is not even brought in for surgical treatment or autopsy unless the owner, or the referring practitioner, so chooses. Again much information available in veterinary pathologic laboratories is never published and even then may be restricted to rare or unusual cases. However, with the advent of indexing and computerized recording, a start is being made to bring such unpublished material to light, as, for example, in Priester's valuable surveys of material in 12 North American veterinary schools.[165]

Although a number of veterinary school studies of animal tumors have been published, their statistical value has been diminished by the absence of information about the background animal population. This situation is being remedied (cf. the Alameda County surveys in California[52-54]). The common practice of spaying cats and the increasingly common practice of spaying bitches will even here distort the true picture of the incidence of uterine and ovarian tumors.

Abattoir surveys are not easy to organize, but they can provide valuable information, as in the case of the federally inspected abattoirs in the United States,[21] the British survey by Anderson, Sandison, and Jarrett,[7] and a recent survey in Australia.[192] It must be remembered that food animals are slaughtered at an early age, in contrast to domestic pets and horses, which are more often allowed to live out something closer to an expected lifespan.

A considerable advance in the study of animal neoplasms was the establishment of the Registry of Veterinary Pathology at the Armed Forces Institute of Pathology in Washington, D.C. Computerized recording of tumors in animals in zoos is also developing,[10] and neoplasms in lower animals are being studied at the Registry of Tumors in the Lower Animals (RTLA) at the Smithsonian Institution, also in Washington, D.C.

A basic need in studying tumors of animals is for some standardized nomenclature, preferably in harmony with that of human neoplasms. The World Health Organization has interested itself in this problem and has recently published[214] its first set of classifications of tumors in six domesticated mammalian species, horse, ox, pig, sheep, dog, and cat. The classification of tumors of the female genital system should appear shortly.[123,161]

Attention may finally be drawn to what might be termed the "negative" significance of studying *spontaneous* tumors in animals. The "positive" significance is clear: A study of tumors occurring commonly in animals may provide epidemiologic or other clues to their etiology,[42] and the tumors provide opportunities for etiologic, biologic, and therapeutic investigation. For example, there is in some stocks of rabbits a high incidence of endometrial glandular tumors, which allows histogenetic and genetic analyses of considerable comparative oncologic interest. The "negative" significance may arise if careful study indicates that certain tumors of importance in humans are rarely if ever seen in animals.[43] For example, the observation that carcinoma of the uterine cervix is reported only very rarely as a spontaneous tumor in animals and that choriocarcinoma is reliably reported even more rarely may add weight to the proposition that factors that are more or less specific to the human patient are involved in the etiology of these particular tumors.

Spontaneous Tumors of the Uterus

In a detailed literature review 10 years ago,[41] I showed that endometrial carcinoma is significant only in cows and rabbits, and that carcinoma of the uterine cervix is rarely encountered in animals. Most examples of bovine uterine carcinoma have been reported in the United States, at least in recent years, and most endometrial tumors of rabbits have been seen in three colonies in that country. In no domesticated species has choriocarcinoma been convincingly diagnosed.

The main part of this section is concerned with endometrial tumors in cows and in rabbits. Before these are dealt with, however, a brief survey is made of uterine tumors in other domesticated animals (horse, sheep, goat, pig, dog, cat, fowl), laboratory animals, and wild and zoo animals and birds.

Domesticated Animals: General Survey

Mare (Equus caballus)

Carcinoma of the uterine corpus or cervix has been rarely recorded in mares, and detailed pathologic reports are lacking. Myometrial tumors may be more important than endometrial tumors. Malignant as well as benign muscle tumors have been encountered. Jennings[41] found a probable leiomyosarcoma in the uterus of a 12-year-old mare, and Grant[79] reported a curious case of a leiomyoma of the right uterine cornu of a 12-year-old thoroughbred mare: The foal present showed extensive deformities of the extremities of all four limbs.

Records of epidermoid carcinoma of the vagina, vulva,[196] and clitoris of the mare are more common. These tumors resemble, in their papilliform structure and slow metastasizing course, the more common epidermoid carcinoma of the glans penis of the castrated male horse, and it is possible that the carcinomas have a common etiology (smegma ?, virus ?) in the two sexes.

Ewe (Ovis aries)

Practically all reported tumors of the genital tract of the ewe have been leiomyomas of the uterus or fibromas of the vagina.[21] There is one report of a probable endometrial carcinoma in a 5-year-old crossbred ewe by Terlecki and Watson,[195] who have found a poorly differentiated mucus-secreting adenocarcinoma of the uterine wall.

Goat (*Capra hircus*)

The total number of tumors of any kind whatever that have been reported in goats is very small. In Kronberger's survey[117] there are listed 24 caprine tumors, which include one fibroma of the uterus, one adenoma of the vagina and vulva, and three fibromas of the vagina and vulva. Riedel[168] reported a sclerosing metastasizing adenocarcinoma in the region of the uterus of a 12-year-old goat that had not been pregnant for some years. Brandly[41] had also seen a caprine uterine adenocarcinoma, and Barboni[41] reported a mucous cystadenocarcinoma of the uterine cervix.

Sow (*Sus scrofa*)

No convincing report of uterine or cervical carcinoma in the sow has come to my notice. Most reported tumors are myomas or fibromas, some affecting the uterus and vagina and some the broad ligament. For example, Winterfeldt[213] found a leiomyoma measuring 53 by 38 by 17 cm and weighing 20.62 kg in the broad ligament of the right cornu of an old sow.

Dog (*Canis familiaris*)

The number of reported cases of adenocarcinoma of the canine uterus is quite small.[41,75] The unwary pathologist may be deceived by the development of hyperplastic glandular changes, which may be quite localized, in cases of the common condition of "pyometra," or by the apparent myometrial invasion in adenomyosis uteri.[34,181] This may be the true diagnosis of the lesion reported as a uterine adenocarcinoma by Joshi et al.[109]

However, acceptable cases of canine endometrial carcinoma are on record. In one case,[5] the tumor affected the right uterine cornu, with metastases in the lungs, bronchial nodes, liver, spleen, pericardium, gastrointestinal tract, kidneys, and pancreas. It is probable that this was a spontaneous tumor but the host, dying at 10 years of age, was a Beagle bitch that, in an experimental lifespan evaluation of the effects of irradiation, had received whole-body exposures of 75 rads each at 7-day intervals at the age of 11 months. The bitch had produced two litters, at 96 and 130 weeks of age, and had shown false estrus or anestrus for 1,300 days before death.

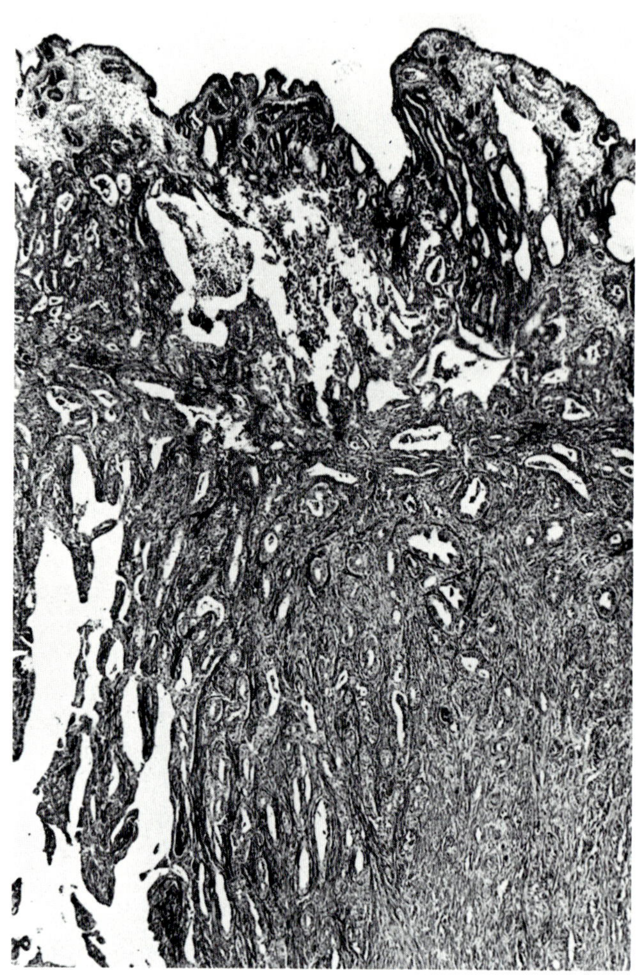

39.1 Adenocarcinoma of the uterus of a 10-year-old Persian cat, showing endometrial origin and deep invasion of myometrium. ×32.

Carcinoma of the uterine cervix seems to be as great a rarity in the bitch as it is in other domesticated mammals. Dämmrich and Lettow[45] reported an adenocarcinoma, possibly arising from cervical glands, in a 14-year-old Dachshund bitch.

There is no convincing record of a choriocarcinoma in a bitch; the most likely example is that recorded by Christopher[33] in a 2½-year-old Alsatian bitch. Two sorts of cell were described in the lesion—large round cells, and syncytial cells—which probably occupied a placental site.

The common tumor of the canine female genital tract is a leiomyoma or other mesodermal tumor of the vagina.[11,127]

In a series of 3,073 tumor-bearing dogs, Brodey and Roszel[22] found 96 tumors of the uterus, vagina, and vulva

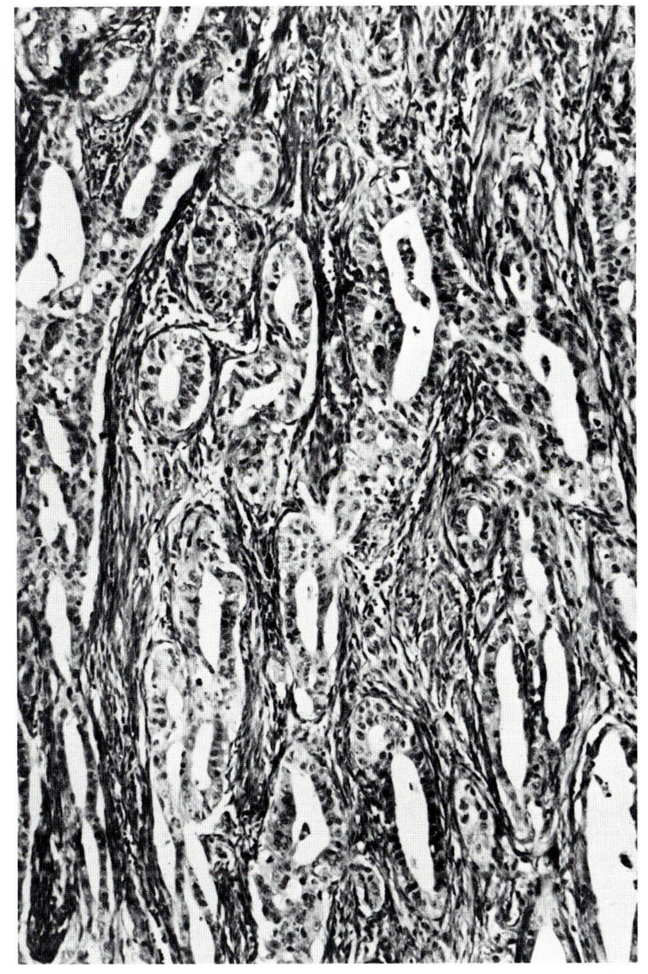

39.2 Same tumor as in Figure 39.1, showing well-differentiated glandular pattern. ×127.

in 90 bitches. The commonest tumor was a leiomyoma, 76 such tumors being found in 70 dogs (66 affecting the vagina and vulva and only 10 the uterus). Affected bitches averaged 10.8 years of age. Most of the myomas affected the vestibule of the vulva, growth being extraluminal or intraluminal. In this series, there were also three leiomyosarcomas.

Cat (*Felis catus*)

Female cats are frequently subjected to ovariohysterectomy. Since my 1964 review, Preiser[164] and Belter, Crawford, and Bates[18] have described endometrial adenocarcinomas in cats, both aged 11 years. I have seen one case of endometrial adenocarcinoma (Figures 39.1 and 39.2), as well as a possible carcinoleiomyosarcoma. O'Rourke and Geib,[157] who state that only eight uterine carcinomas have been recorded in cats, described a case in a 12-year-old domestic short-haired cat. Dystocia was noted 2 months previously. One month later a blackish green vaginal discharge developed. The cat showed incoordination, and there was bilateral retinal hemorrhage and detachment. Metastases from the endometrial carcinoma were found in the ovaries, adrenal, lung, brain, and eyes.

Squamous cell carcinoma of the uterine cervix seems to be as rare in cats as in other domesticated animals, but squamous metaplasia may be found in some endometrial carcinomas.[139]

Fowl (*Gallus domesticus*)

Although the fowl oviduct differs structurally and functionally from the mammalian uterus, it is worth drawing attention to the remarkable incidence of carcinoma of the oviduct that has recently been encountered in the United Kingdom. Goodchild and Cooper,[77] for example, in a flock of Light Sussex hens 66 to 68 weeks old, found that 84 (37.7%) of 223 birds examined had macroscopic tumors in the magnum of the single (left) oviduct. Metastases were noted macroscopically in three hens.

The tumor is diffuse or nodular and is generally multifocal in origin, being more pronounced toward the cranial end of the oviduct.[76] It affects active and regressed oviducts and it can affect the normally nonpersistent right oviduct.

Laboratory Animals: General Survey

Primates

In their survey of tumors in nonhuman primates, O'Gara and Adamson[156] stated that 41 tumors of female sex organs have been reported in 39 primates.

In a survey of neoplasms and proliferative lesions in 1,065 nonhuman primate necropsies, Seibold and Wolf[182] recorded leiomyoma of the uterus in three *Pan troglodytes* (aged 23, 44, and over 44 years, respectively) and in two *Macaca mulatta* (both adult, one multiparous). An old multiparous *M. mulatta* showed adenomatous hyperplasia of the endocervical glands, developing in the everted mucosa of the posterior lip of the cervix and the posterior fornix. Seibold and Wolf also refer to six cases (in 317 female *M. mulatta*) of endometriosis, or extrauterine occurrence of tissue resembling the uterine mucous membrane. One monkey, killed after signs of abdominal distress, showed intestinal adhesions from endometrial proliferations in the peritoneal cavity.

An account of endometriosis in rhesus monkeys is given by McCann and Myers.[138] Twenty-one of 69 mature females examined had such lesions, which increased in incidence with parity, age, increasing number of hysterotomies, and increased time since last pregnancy. The lesions are described and their incidence analyzed in detail, and it is concluded that "there exist basic differences in the pathogenesis and the pattern of pathology of this disease in the monkey as compared to that in man. It would thus appear that theories of pathogenesis of this disease valid for monkey may not necessarily be valid for man" (p. 583).

Recently, Strozier et al.[190] have described lesions in a female *M. mulatta,* approximately 15 years old, that died after an extended period of diarrhea and weight loss. At autopsy, there were found cystic endometrial hyperplasia and foci of endometrial tissue in the uterine wall, colon, and a regional lymph node. A focus of adenocarcinoma was found in the proliferated endometrium. The endometrial cavity contained purulent fluid from which a pure culture of *Escherichia coli* was isolated.

Special mention may be made of the metastasizing cervical carcinoma that Hisaw and Hisaw[96] found in an old female *M. mulatta,* and the cervical carcinoma *in situ* that Sternberg[185] found in a young adult of the same species.

Digiacomo and McCann[51] also found a case of carcinoma *in situ* of the cervix in one of 63 female *M. mulatta.* Hertig and MacKey[94] examined the complete genital tracts of 11 adult female crab-eating monkeys, *M. fascicularis,* and the same number of adult chimpanzees, *Pan troglodytes.* In one of the monkeys, a mature individual whose endometrium was in the preovulatory phase, the cervix showed an extensive squamous cell carcinoma *in situ,* involving the ventral portion of the glandular mucosa of the inner endocervix and the outer endocervix, the area most exposed to the vaginal environment in this species. There was no histologic contiguity with the normal squamous epithelium of the exocervix (the endocervix and the exocervix in this species are separated by an encircling fornix). Eight of the other 10 monkeys showed squamous metaplasia of the endocervix or of the exocervix or (in two animals) of both. One of the chimpanzees, 22 to 23 years old, showed three leiomyomas of the uterine fundus and corpus. In sections of endomyometrium of the corpus there were changes classified as proliferative endometrium, a focus of adenomatous hyperplasia, and a focus of adenocarcinoma *in situ.*

Moreland and Woodard[144] described a possible uterine hamartoma in an adult cottontop marmoset [*Saguinus* (*Oepomidas*) *oedipus*]. Of particular interest is the report by Lindsey et al.[121] of what they considered to be the only reported case of choriocarcinoma in a nonhuman primate. A rhesus monkey became pregnant in the laboratory. It was subsequently given norethindrone enanthate daily except at weekends for 1 month, but it is not thought that this was involved in the occurrence of the tumor. The monkey died, but no fetus was found in the uterus, which contained a thick yellow material with ragged brown fragments. A large uterine mass was diagnosed as a choriocarcinoma, with extensive metastases in the lungs. In the trophoblastic tumor, cells of cytotrophoblast predominated. Granulomatous lesions, possibly tuberculous, were superimposed on the lung lesions.

In passing, mention may be made of the choriocarcinoma found in a pregnant nine-banded armadillo,[133] which had been given 100 mg thalidomide per kilogram of body weight per day for 10 days and was killed 17 days after the first dose. This mammal possesses a hemochorial placenta which resembles that of man in its maternal–fetal border.

Mouse

Spontaneous carcinomas and sarcomas of the mouse uterus[175] have been reported by a few authors.[41] Age-related uterine leiomyomas or leiomyosarcomas were studied by Malinin and Malinin[132] and Chouroulinkov, Guillon, and Guérin[31] surveyed 130 cases of endometrial sarcomas. Gardner and Pan[72] found 13 of 56 female mice of Pybus Miller stock, 200 days old or older, had cervical or vaginal tumors at the time of death (five carcinomas of the vagina or uterine cervix, seven probably of epithelial origin, and one spindle cell sarcoma).

Rat

A variety of uterine tumors[41,175] has been reported in rats, including adenocarcinomas and sarcomas (some of which were leiomyosarcomas). The tumors are not very frequently encountered but sometimes they achieve a moderate importance. For example, Schulze[180] found 23 uterine carcinomas among 34 spontaneous tumors of the uterus and ovaries in 66 tumors in 1,373 autopsied Sprague–Dawley and Bethesda Black rats.

Recent reports include those by Snell,[184] Jacobs and Huseby,[106] and Schardein *et al.*[177] In rats examined in the Laboratory of Pathology of the National Cancer Institute Snell[184] recorded that nearly two-thirds of the animals of F344 strain and one-third of those of the M520 strain over

20 months of age had endometrial tumors. Only a few OM, ACI, and BUF rats had similar tumors, and none were found in WN rats. In the strains with high incidence, but not in others, the tumors were more often found in virgins than in breeders. Most of the tumors were adenomatous polyps, a few were angiosarcomas. One BUF and two ACI rats showed endometrial adenocarcinomas, and one BUF rat had a uterine horn, lined with squamous cells, and showing two foci of squamous cell carcinoma. One 24-month-old F344 rat had a uterine myoma. The only cervical tumor noted was a polyp in a 27-month-old OM breeder. Yang[218] recorded a remarkable keratinizing metaplasia in a virgin 22-month-old Sprague–Dawley rat—one cornu (right) was completely affected, whereas the other showed only two microscopic foci.

Jacobs and Huseby[106] found macroscopic tumors of the uterine horns in 21 of 95 autopsied female Fischer rats. They occurred at an average age of 669 days, including some rats less than 1 year old. The tumors, often multiple, were polypoid glandular structures, mostly covered by endometrial epithelium. One consisted of very cellular sarcomatous tissue and three others showed sarcomatous change. All four sarcomas were transplanted, as were five benign polyps. It was concluded that the sarcomas were not of smooth muscle origin but arose from the lamina propria of the endometrial polyps. Schardein, Fitzgerald, and Kaump[177] found four Holtzman-source rats with well-differentiated adenomatous endometrial polyps with an average latent period of 467 days. Thompson et al.[199] have described similar tumors in a 2-year-old Sprague–Dawley rat, as well as cases of leiomyosarcoma of the uterus and fibrovascular polyp of the cervix.

Gellatly[74] has drawn attention to the need for histologic study in the diagnosis of uterine tumors in rats—a misdiagnosis of pyometra can occur. In a series of some 50 25-month-old virgin Wistar rats, the uterus was the organ most often affected by tumors; half the tumors were fibroadenomas, the next most common being a highly malignant adenocarcinoma. Some tumors were squamous cell carcinomas, which could sometimes be traced to originate from preexisting areas of squamous metaplasia of the endometrium (present in 28% of this series of rats), and in a few animals such metaplasia, with squamous cell carcinoma formation, was found on the surface of a fibroadenoma.

Guinea pig

Lipschutz et al.[124] found two leiomyomas of the uterus in animals over 5 years of age, and two (histologic) adenocarcinomas in animals $3\frac{1}{2}$ and 5 years old. Rogers and Blumenthal[172] listed the following uterine tumors: four fibro- and leiomyomas, one adenomyoma, three fibro- and leiomyosarcomas, and one mesenchymal mixed tumor.

Hamster

In a colony of Chinese hamsters (*Cricetulus griseus*) Ward and Moore[204] found uterine tumors in 30 of 120 females. These were adenocarcinomas, firm whitish nodular growths that always appeared to have included the cervical area, although they did not necessarily originate in the cervix. Implantations were not infrequent on visceral and parietal peritoneum, and three animals showed lung secondaries when examined histologically. The lesions showed extensive stromal fibrosis. The tumors usually occurred in the second year of life. The authors refer to a personal communication from Yerganian who stated that the incidence of such lesions could be enhanced by radiation.

Gerbil

Rowe et al.[173] found 44 neoplasms at necropsy in 37 of 115 gerbils from a colony which contained wild-caught and first or second generation laboratory-raised gerbils (mostly *Meriones* species). The tumors included a moderately differentiated adenocarcinoma of the oviduct in *M. lybicus,* and endometrial adenocarcinoma in *M. tristrami* and the *M. shawi* × *M. lybicus* hybrid. (Both these latter animals also had granulosa cell tumors of the ovary.) Two other gerbils (*M. shawi* and *Pachyuromys duprisi*) had uterine leiomyosarcomas.

Wild Animals, Animals in Zoos, and Birds: General Survey

In her impressive bibliographic survey of references to diseases in wild and zoo mammals and birds, Halloran[90] includes references to the following tumors of the uterus:

Fibroma: armadillo, agouti, axis deer, yak, nylghaie, blesbok, antelope
Fibroid: agouti, black leopard, lion, elephant
Fibromyoma: squirrel, lion
Myoma: lion, elephant
Carcinoma: coypu, mink, lion, wild swine, bontebok, gemsbok, sable antelope

Other tumors of the uterus referred to include: chorionic epithelioma and chorioma in porcupines; uterine tumor in an aardwolf; adenoma of cervix in the lion; cystic tumor in the jaguar; fibroadenoma in a jaguar. A tumor of the oviduct in Psittaciformes is listed. "A tumor was reported in the vagina of a hyena" (p. 200).

A female gray seal, shot at an estimated age of 44 years, had uterine squamous cell carcinomas and leiomyomas.[137]

Rewell and Willis[167] examined a uterine fibromyoma, 4 cm across, from a whale.

Domesticated Animals: Detailed Account

Attention may now be concentrated on the two species in which uterine endometrial adenocarcinoma has been encountered in significant numbers—the cow and the rabbit.

Cow (Bos taurus)

Although carcinoma of the bovine uterus has been recorded in a number of countries,[41,111,142,201] it is noteworthy that in recent years the majority of such tumors have been encountered in cows in federally inspected abattoirs in the United States. There is a strong possibility that such tumors are overlooked in many abattoirs elsewhere, since butchers commonly discard the uterus after only the most casual inspection. However, even in the careful abattoir survey by Anderson and Sandison[6] of tumors encountered in 1.3 million cattle at abattoirs in Great Britain, no tumors of the uterine corpus or cornu were found (there were three squamous cell carcinomas of the cervix in cows 6 to 8 years old). A search is still worth making—I have recently examined a metastasizing bovine uterine adenocarcinoma from a London abattoir.

The key papers on bovine uterine adenocarcinoma are those based on findings in American abattoirs.[21,141,143] In fact, these tumors are almost always abattoir findings. A clinical case was described by Lingard and Dickinson:[122] A 4-year-old Hereford cow with metastases in the lungs, liver, and bronchial, mediastinal, and internal iliac nodes was pregnant with a 100-day fetus in the right cornu, which showed, on its lesser curvature, a firm discoid carcinoma, 8 by 3 cm. That uterine carcinoma is not incompatible with pregnancy in cows has long been known. Wyssmann[216] found an affected cow with twin calves, and three of the 79 cases of Migaki et al.[141] were pregnant. This is consistent with the observation that the ovaries and the nonneoplastic endometrium showed no significant deviation from normal cyclic changes in the cows examined by Monlux et al.[143]

The relative incidence of bovine uterine carcinoma in American abattoirs is indicated by Brandly and Migaki.[21]

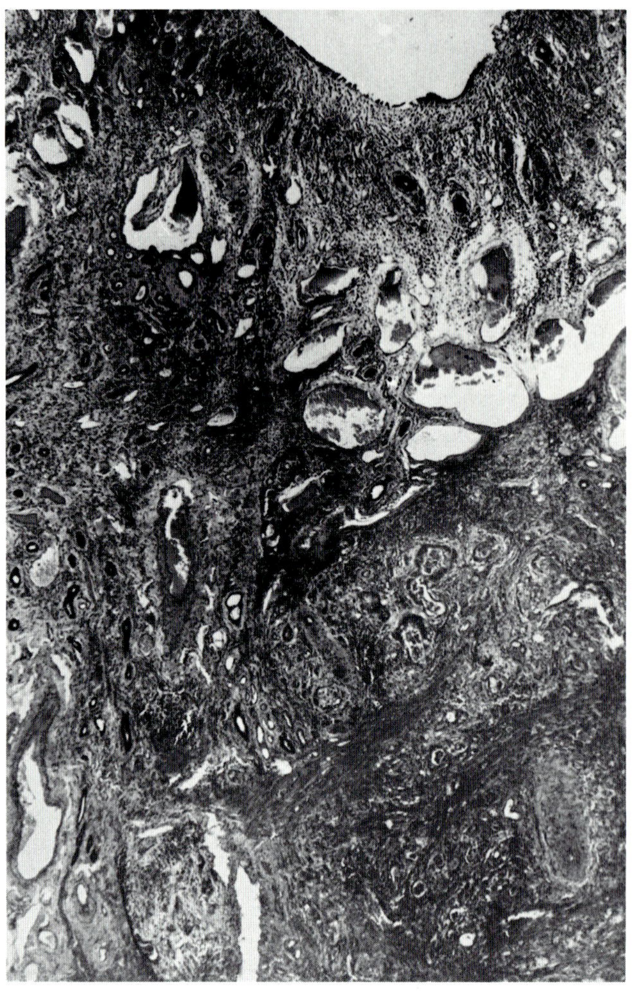

39.3 Adenocarcinoma of the uterus of an 11-year-old cow, showing deep origin in endometrium. Metastases were present in regional nodes, lungs, kidney, heart, bronchial, and mediastinal nodes. ×32.

[From a section kindly provided by Dr. George Migaki (4004-AFIP 1448288).]

In a total of 737 tumors of all kinds (484 malignant, 253 benign) examined in less than 10 years, this was the second most common tumor submitted for histologic examination—lymphosarcoma 177, uterine carcinoma 166.

Affected cows[141] range from 2 to 12 years of age, most being over 6 years. There is no indication of breed susceptibility. The carcinoma is usually a single lesion, although occasionally two or three separate primary tumors may be present. The lesion is generally located in the free rather than the common part (body) of the uterine horns. It is generally firm and fibrous; white, whitish-yellow, or yel-

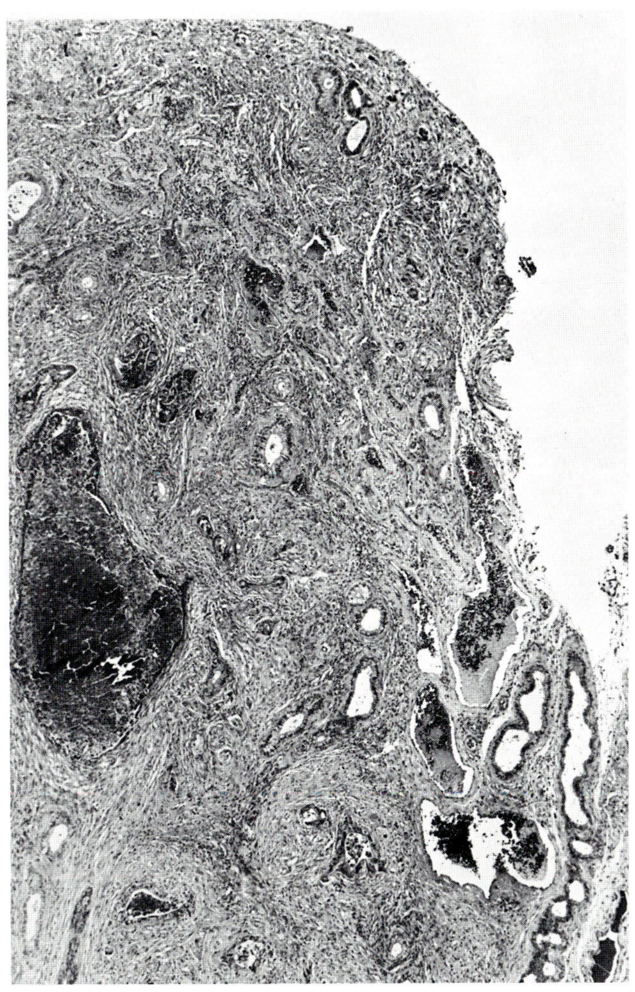

39.4 Adenocarcinoma of the uterus of a cow from London abattoir, showing endometrial tumor. ×32.

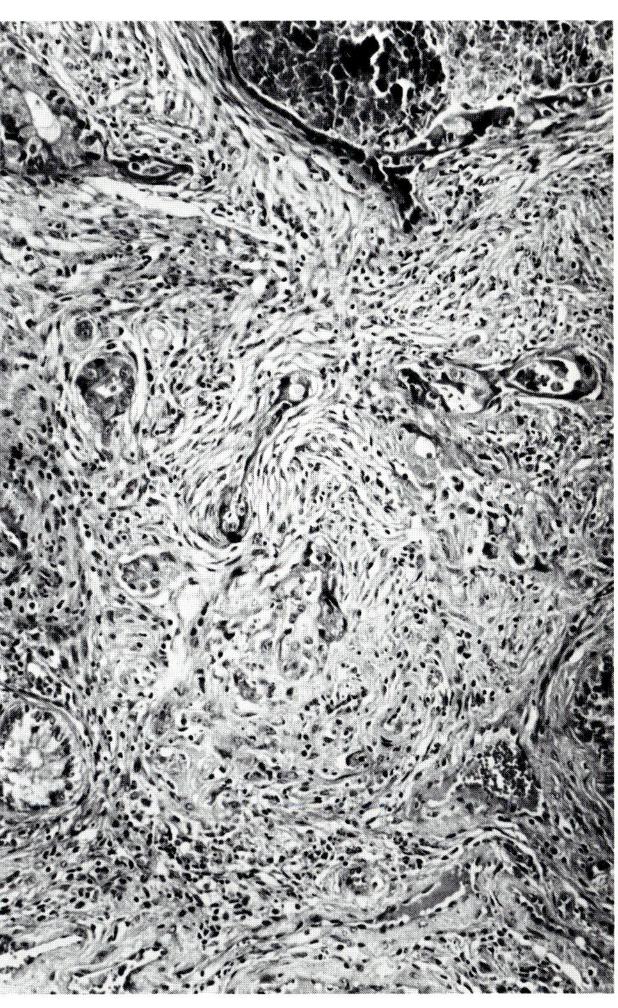

39.5 Same tumor as Figure 39.4, showing sclerosing primary endometrial carcinoma. ×127.

low; and sometimes calcified. Small tumors can easily be overlooked. The thickening of the wall is rather diffuse and may be outwardly umbilicated. The tumor appears to develop deep in the endometrium (Figures 39.3 and 39.4) and the endometrial and serosal surfaces may appear grossly uninvolved. The tumor is typically accompanied by the abundant formation of dense fibrous tissue (Figure 39.5), which may lead to the incorrect diagnosis of sarcoma or even of mixed tumor. The tendency to marked sclerosis is also a feature of metastases, but in them the glandular conformation is usually retained (Figure 39.6).

The endometrial tumor extends locally to the serosa and the ovaries, this being accompanied by the local formation of a dense mat of fibrous tissue, the presence of which, as Trotter[200] recognized, as an abattoir finding, points strongly to the presence of a uterine carcinoma. The visceral and parietal peritoneum may show neoplastic spread, especially near the uterus, and metastases may be found in the nodes and viscera. In one series of 26 cases, Monlux et al.[143] found metastases in lung (22), bronchial node (12), mediastinal node (14), sublumbar node (15), internal iliac node (17), and ovary (5), as well as on peritoneal surfaces. The metastatic growths, in lymph nodes particularly, are firm, white, or yellow and may be calcified; they therefore resemble granulomas, such as tuberculosis. Once pulmonary deposits have formed, they may increase in number by local "closed-circuit" lymphatic–vascular spread.

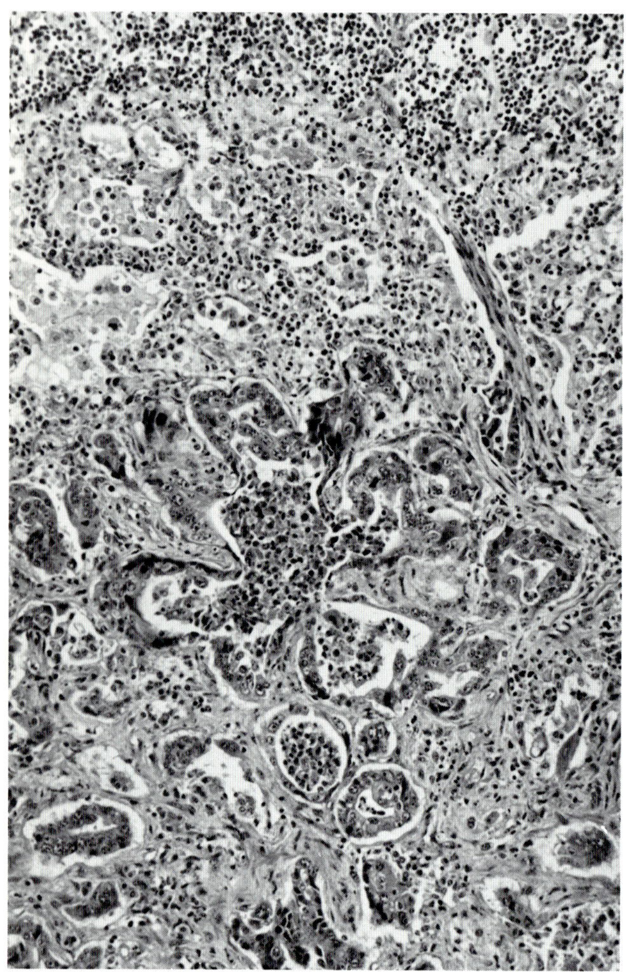

39.6 Same tumor as Figure 39.4, showing retention of glandular conformation in a pulmonary metastasis. ×127.

Since Ottosen[160] suggested that the uterus might be an important site of origin for deposits of adenocarcinoma metastases in the bovine lung, Monlux et al.[143] have carefully described the histology of pulmonary metastases of known primary uterine adenocarcinomas in cows, stressing their retention of differentiated structure and the marked fibrous sclerosis. Hartigan and Flynn[93] in Eire have described pulmonary lesions in a cow that fulfilled these histologic criteria for a carcinoma of uterine origin. (In passing, it is worth noting that the bovine endometrium is sometimes the site of lymphosarcoma.)

Few cases of uterine cervical carcinoma have been described in cows.[6,41]

A variety of other tumors have been reported in the bovine female genital tract, including leiomyomas, fibromas, and fibromyomas. Most of these occur in the vaginal wall. My own series of vaginal tumors[38] included seven fibromas, seven lipomas, three fibromyomas, and two leiomyomas. Some uterine myomas may become fantastically large; Vandeplasche and Thoonen[202] recorded a weight of 200 kg. Some smooth muscle tumors are malignant. Maeda et al.[130] found a leiomyosarcoma of low-grade malignancy. Noordsy et al.[150] reported a leiomyosarcoma of the uterus in an 8-year-old Holstein cow, with secondaries on the omentum, diaphragm, and peritoneum and in the mesenteric lymph nodes, lungs, pleura, and myocardium. The primary tumor measured 75 by 50 by 30 cm and (together with the uterus) weighed 75 kg. The lesion in an extirpated uterine mass (weighing 110 kg) reported by Keindorf[113] was a partially cartilaginous mesenchymal tumor. It is not known whether uterine mixed tumors occur in cows.

Mention should be made of a curious vascular mesenchymal lesion of the bovine fetal placenta, which has been called a "choriohemangioma." Karlson and Kelly[112] found such a lesion in a 2-year-old cow that had given birth to a healthy calf. The lesion, attached to the fetal surface of the allantochorion by a narrow pedicle, measured 6 by 3 by 3 cm. It was the only such lesion found in a study of 550 membranes. Drieux and Le Coustumier[56] found a similar but larger lesion in a 3-year-old Montbéliard cow. A still larger tumor (30 by 20 by 7.5 cm) was examined by Corcoran and Murphy:[35] The fourth calf of a 6-year-old crossbred Hereford cow, a male, was born alive, followed by the tumor, composed of capillaries in a loose embryonal stroma. This lesion was accompanied by a remarkable degree of hydramnios. That such placental tumors are hamartomas rather than true neoplasms is supported by the observation by Kirkbride, Bicknell, and Robl[115] of a lesion of the placenta of a cow, when the calf, aborted at about 8 months gestation, showed angiomatous masses of the skin of the left forelimb and on the ventrolateral surface of the tongue.

Laboratory Animal: Detailed Account

Rabbit (*Oryctolagus cuniculus*)

There are several reports of uterine endometrial epithelial tumors in rabbits.[41] Greene[84] has summarized his outstanding pioneer work on these tumors, and a valuable illustrated summary account is given by Weisbroth.[207] Their value as animal models for the study of human endometrial adenocarcinomas has been discussed by Baba and von Haam.[13] The tumors have been reported in

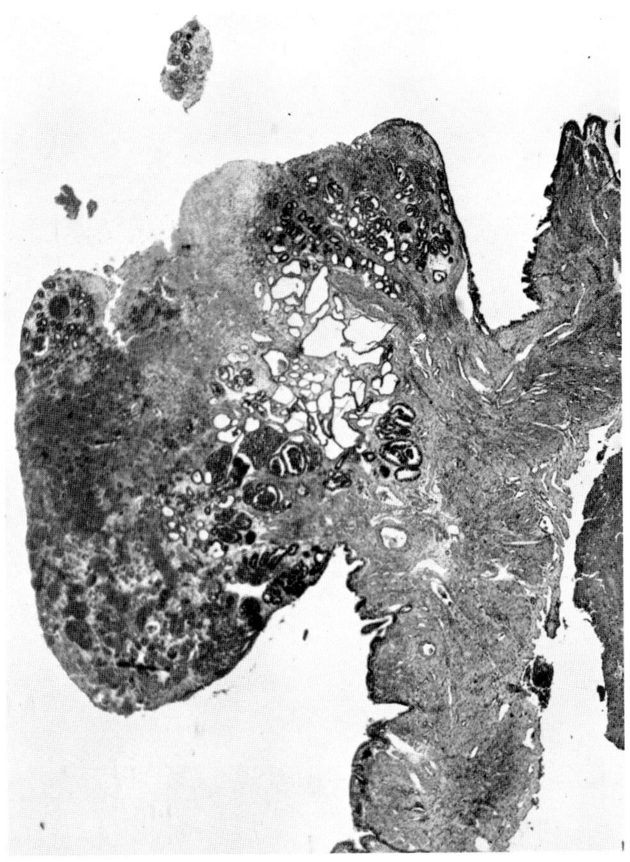

39.7 Adenocarcinoma of the uterus of a rabbit, showing polypoid endometrial tumor with invasion of myometrium. ×25.

[Photograph kindly provided by the Imperial Cancer Research Fund, Tumor Reference Collection 145, Polson's case.]

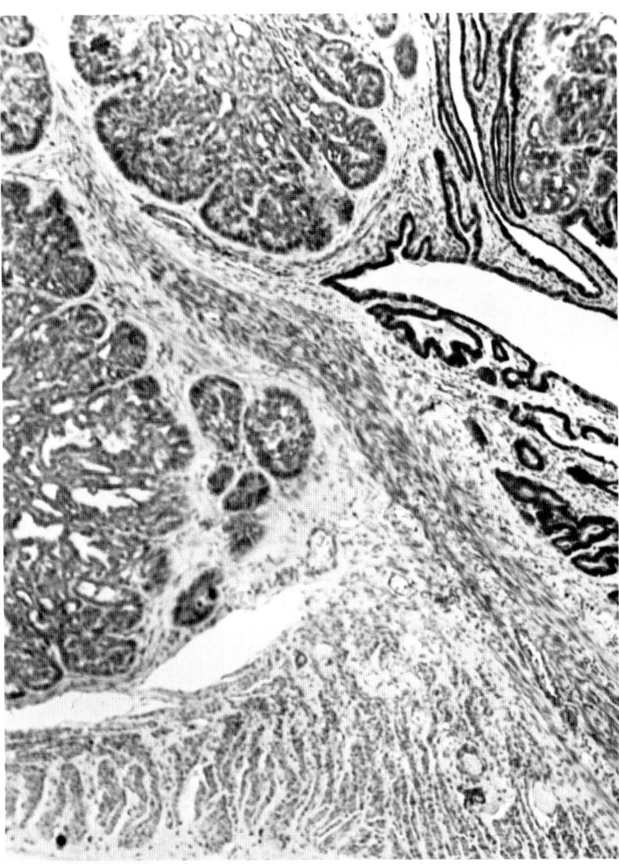

39.8 Adenocarcinoma of the uterus of a rabbit, showing morphology and myometrial invasion. ×108.

[Photograph kindly provided by the Imperial Cancer Research Fund, Tumor Reference Collection 145, Polson's case.]

Europe (Figures 39.7 and 39.8) as well as America, but most of them have been in three rabbit colonies: those studied by Greene and his colleagues in the Rockefeller Institute rabbitry following a move from New York to Princeton; those in the Henry Phipps Institute colony of the University of Pennsylvania, studied by Ingalls et al.[102]; and those in the Dutch rabbits in the Ohio State University colony, studied by Baba and von Haam themselves. As summarized by Baba and von Haam,[13] Greene and his colleagues found 142 adenomas and adenocarcinomas of the endometrium in a colony of 849 rabbits observed for 9 years. Ingalls et al. found 353 uterine tumors in 1,735 rabbits in a colony observed for 30 years. Baba and von Haam[13] found 16 adenocarcinomas (two *in situ*) in the uteruses of 83 out of 117 Dutch rabbits studied for 30 months.

The salient feature of uterine endometrial tumors in rabbits is that they tend to occur with increasing frequency in older animals.[102] Burrows[25] found that 50% of his noninbred rabbits surviving to the age of 2½ years had endometrial tumors, and such tumors may occur in animals 7 or even 9 years of age.

In the Rockefeller Institute colony, following its move from New York to Princeton,[80] Greene and Saxton[87] found 83 rabbits with uterine endometrial tumors—adenomas and adenocarcinomas were not readily distinguishable—in a colony of about 500 breeding does in a 4-year period. Eight of the rabbits died of metastases. The tumors were discovered, either by palpation or at autopsy, at an average age of 45 months. They were confined to breeding females but disturbances of reproductive function, such as reduction of litter size, fertility, and maternal care, preceded the detection and probably the initiation of the tumors. The early lesions were either single or often multiple and might affect one or both horns. They appeared as pedunculated growths, or small thickenings of the endometrium, usually on the endometrial folds adjacent to the mesometrial insertion. The tumors might remain small or reach the size of a hen's egg in 6 months. Metastases were somewhat delayed, considering the early signs of vascular invasion, but they were found in all cases in which the known duration of the tumor was over 1 year. A possibly significant observation was, that prior to metastasis, the primary tumor might undergo obvious regressive changes.

Greene,[83] noting the similar breed susceptibility to uterine tumors and to what he called "toxaemia of pregnancy,"[80,81] suggested that liver damage associated with this condition (of unknown origin) might lead to failure by that organ to inactivate estrogen, and this could result in tumor formation. Indeed, histologic alterations that Greene noted in the thyroid, adrenal, pituitary, and mammary glands of the affected rabbits were similar to those seen in estrogen-treated mice, and Meissner et al.[140] have indeed described the experimental production of uterine adenocarcinoma in rabbits by the administration of estrogen. Greene[82] and Greene and Saxton[87] were able to transplant the uterine tumors auto-, homo-, and heterologously (guinea pig eye), but such tumors were not accompanied by the pituitary, thyroid, or adrenal changes accompanying the primary tumors, suggesting that these changes were an indication of the cause rather than the result of the tumors. Greene and Newton[85] showed that the morphologic and transplantation characteristics of the tumors progressed from nonmalignant to malignant states.

Ingalls et al.[102] surveyed the incidence of uterine tumors found by autopsy, abdominal palpation, or laparotomy in the Henry Phipps rabbit colony. They concluded that the dominant factor in the development of uterine carcinomas in these rabbits was age: Of animals dead at 2½ to 3 years of age 8.8% had tumors, whereas of those over 4 years old at death about 60% had tumors. Although there was no significant difference in tumor incidence in breeding and nonbreeding females, there was a difference in strains that had been bred for increased susceptibility to tuberculosis. The possibility that a virus might be involved is mentioned.

Further interesting reports on rabbit endometrial adenocarcinoma, this time in the Ohio State University rabbit colony, are given by Baba and von Haam.[13] Here again, the incidence of tumors increased with age. No association was noted with cystic or glandular endometrial hyperplasia and, in fact, administration of estrogen to aged Dutch

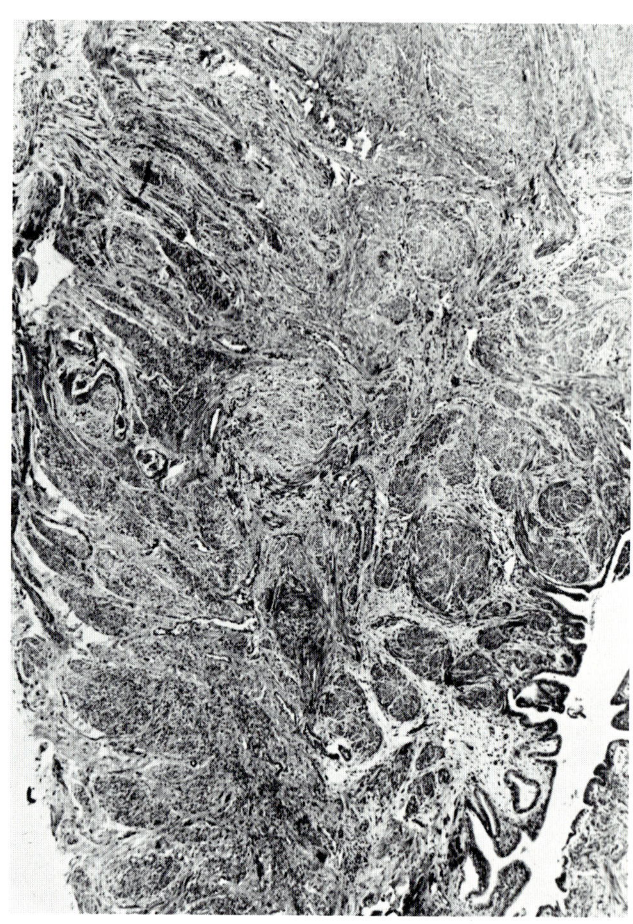

39.9 Leiomyosarcoma of the uterus of a domestic rabbit. ×32.

rabbits reduced the incidence of endometrial carcinomas from 17 to 3%. The tumors were shown by electron microscopy[12] to contain cells resembling those of the deeper endometrial glands.

In commenting on the value of the rabbit endometrial carcinoma as an animal model for the study of the human tumor, Baba and von Haam[13] mentioned that the three major rabbit colonies concerned were no longer maintained. However, they noted that rabbits of the Dutch breed, which they found to be susceptible to such tumors, are commercially available and that investigators could expect to find a number of uterine tumors developing within 1 to 2 years. It is of interest too that the endometrial carcinoma reported by Flatt[67] occurred in an adult multiparous New Zealand rabbit killed for meat purposes. Lombard's[126] three cases in France were in white Angora rabbits.

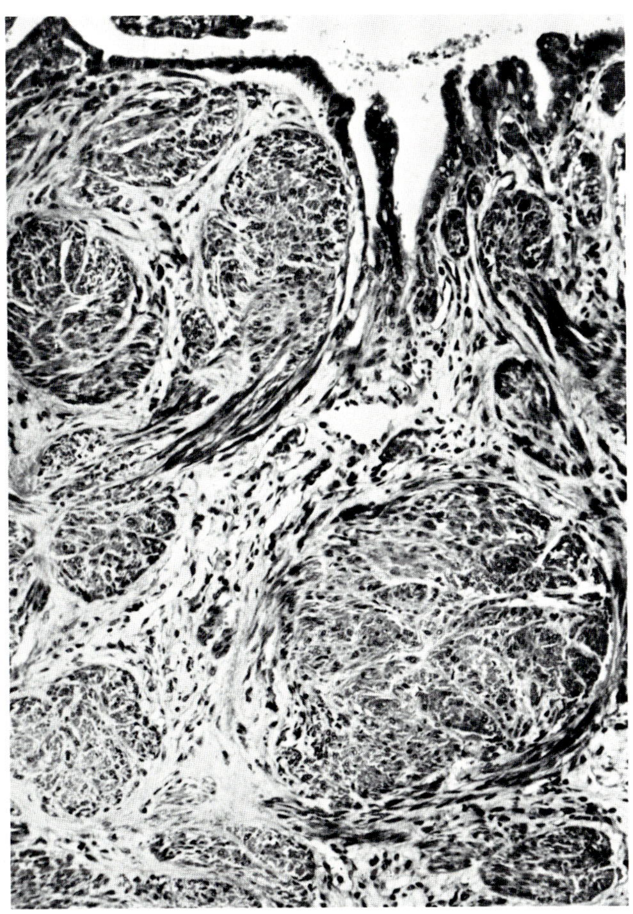

39.10 Same tumor as Figure 39.9, showing multiple origin of the tumor in the myometrium. ×127.

Not all uterine tumors in rabbits are epithelial in nature. Greene and Strauss[88] showed that their uterine carcinomas might be accompanied by uterine myomas and myosarcomas, and Polson[163] and Baba and von Haam[13] also found myosarcomas. I too have seen a metastasizing uterine myosarcoma (Figures 39.9 and 39.10).

Greene, Newton, and Fisk[86] found three cases of squamous cell carcinomas of the columnar–squamous epithelial junction in the vagina of rabbits (all three animals also had uterine carcinomas).

Spontaneous Tumors of the Ovary

Neoplasms of the ovary[161] have been mostly encountered in the cow, the bitch, and the domestic fowl and to a lesser extent in the mare and the cat. The few examples of ovarian tumors in species other than these five will be briefly referred to in domesticated animals (ewe, goat, sow, buffalo), laboratory animals (nonhuman primates, mouse, rat, guinea pig, hamster, gerbil, ferret), and wild animals. The abbreviation GCT will be used throughout for granulosa cell tumor(s). For an account of the comparative morphology of the mammalian ovary see Mossman and Duke.[146]

Domesticated Animals with Infrequently Reported Tumors

Ewe

Neoplasms of the ovary of sheep are rarely recorded. Anderson and Sandison,[6] in their abattoir survey of tumors from 4.5 million sheep in Great Britain, found none and Brandly and Migaki,[21] in their United States abattoir material, found only one, a teratoma. The tumor described by Di Domizio[50] as an arrhenoblastoma could well be a Sertoliform GCT.

Goat

No reference to ovarian tumors in goats has been noted, apart from the "ovarioblastoma sarcomatodes" reported by Hilsdorf,[95] a tumor of uncertain nature.

Sow

According to Nelson et al.,[149] Dobberstein stated that of 188 recorded porcine neoplasms, 18 affected the ovary: 10 cystadenomas, five sarcomas, two teratomas, and one fibroma. They refer to other records of cavernous hemangioma and cystadenocarcinoma and report two hemangiomas (in 52,000 sows), one papillary cystadenoma, and one case of bilateral GCT. The report of hemangioma is interesting, for Maeda et al.[131] found two sows (multiparous Berkshire–Yorkshire cross) with ovarian hemangiomas, and Davis et al.[46] found one. In their abattoir survey in Great Britain, Anderson and Sandison[6] recorded two serous cystadenomas, one GCT, and one leiomyoma. Lombard and Havet[129] saw bilateral metastasizing tumors in a 5-year-old Large White sow. They illustrate the lesion, which they designate "seminoma," but this is in any case a difficult diagnosis to substantiate. The lesion reported as an arrhenoblastoma in a 3-year-old pig by Guarda[89] is more likely to be an abdominal testis in a hermaphrodite. The head-sized "fibromyxosarcoma" of the left ovary of a 9-month-old sow reported by

Schlegel[179] was apparently diagnosed from macroscopic appearance only.

Buffalo

Polding and Lall[162] found teratomas containing hairs in the ovary of four buffaloes.

Laboratory Animals

Primates

A few previously reported ovarian tumors in subhuman primates are tabulated by Martin et al.[134] and by Kraemer and Vera Cruz.[116] Martin et al. themselves report a papillary serous cystadenoma, histologically of low-grade malignancy; a benign cystic teratoma (dermoid cyst); and a cavernous hemangioma. These three cases were found among approximately 75 animals subjected to one or more laparotomies or to autopsy over a 5-year period. The teratoma was in a female that had received 50 rads or less of x irradiation, which was thought to be unlikely to have been of etiologic significance in relation to the dermoid cyst.

The ultrastructural features of a surface papilloma and serous cystadenofibroma, respectively, found incidentally in the ovaries of a 2-year-old rhesus monkey were described by Amin et al.[4] The papilloma contained many ciliated epithelial cells, similar to those of the oviduct epithelium; nonciliated cells resembled the celomic covering of the ovary. In the cystadenoma, there were secretory, ciliated, and "peg" cells, like those of the oviduct epithelium.

Seibold and Wolf,[182] in their series of 1,065 nonhuman primate necropsies, found one case of ovarian adenocarcinoma in an adult *Cebus albifrons;* there was extensive peritoneal implantation. Crews et al.[44] found a mixed lesion, dermoid cyst and papillary cystadenoma, in a young adult rhesus monkey. Weston[209] referred in passing to a thecoma. Rewell[166] found bilateral GCT (and uterine fibromas) in a senile squirrel monkey (*Saimiri sciurea*) that had been in the Lister Institute in London for at least 20 years.

Mouse

A range of tumor types occurs sporadically in the ovary of the mouse.[98,175] In a period of about 15 years, in the Chester Beatty stock mice, 18 ovarian tumors were found[28] in about 3,000 female mice: 13 GCT, two adenocarcinomas, one cystadenoma, one teratoma, and one fibrosarcoma. Some have been found to be transplantable, as with the GCT in a CBA mouse demonstrated by Strong, Gardner, and Hill.[189] Whiteley and Horton[210] found a transplantable hormonally inactive GCT in a 2¼-year-old CBA mouse. A spontaneous carcinoma in the ovary of a C3H mouse was transplantable intraperitoneally[63] into C3HeB/FeJ mice and proved useful in demonstrating the role of lymphatic obstruction in the diaphragm in the development of ascites. C3HeB mice have been studied particularly by Deringer,[48] who found mainly GCT and tubular adenomas but also luteomas and a mixed tumor. She quotes Woolley and Little as having seen a 33% incidence of ovarian tumors in strain CE mice, and Dickie as noting a 52% incidence of ovarian tumors in CE backcross mice. Bielschowsky and d'Ath[20] have drawn attention to what may be a suitable animal model of GCT, which occurred with some frequency in three of four inbred strains of mice they studied in New Zealand. In mice surviving the age of the first tumor-bearing animals, routine histologic sectioning of ovaries revealed GCT in NZC (virgins, 15 out of 45; breeders, eight out of 39), NZO (virgins, nine out of 199; breeders, seven out of 45) and NZY (virgins, three out of 82; breeders, four out of 183), but no such tumors were found in NZB mice, whose median age was lower than for the other three strains. The two chief tumor patterns were cylindromatous and follicular. Eight tumors were classified as diffuse (malignant). The tumors in NZO mice appeared to be nonfunctional, and although hyperplasia of the endometrium was present in each NZC tumor-bearing mouse, cystic endometrial hyperplasia was present in practically all animals in the second year of life. Gardner, Strong, and Smith[73] in a 695-day-old Strong E1 mouse, found a chromophobe adenoma of the pituitary, bilateral ovarian GCT, endometrial hyperplasia, and multiple, small mammary adenocarcinomas. Hooker and Strong[97] found a GCT in a hermaphrodite.

Jackson and Brues[105] found an embryoma in a C3H mouse which could be transplanted subcutaneously, intrasplenically, and intrahepatically. Fawcett[58] found bilateral ovarian teratomas in a Swiss mouse, and Fekete and Ferrigno[62] reported a transplantable teratoma in a C3H mouse (see also Thiery[197]). Scheuler and Ediger[178] found a unilateral teratoma of the ovary in a C3H/HeN clinically normal breeder mouse. They illustrate a focus of epithelial cells suggestive of malignant transformation.

Particular interest attaches to the reports[147,148,174] of the development of tubular adenomas of the ovary of mice of the (C57Bl/6J × C3H/HeJ) F_1 W^x/W^x genotype. Such mice have few oocytes at birth, and their number

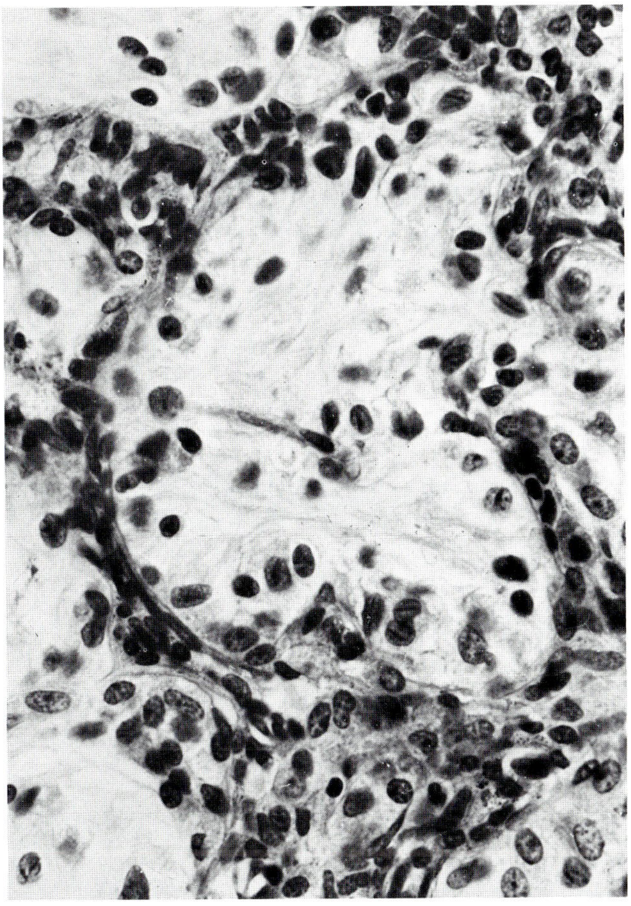

39.11 Rat ovary, showing Sertoliform tubules. Note "grooved" nuclei. ×813.

[From a section kindly provided by D. S. G. Patton.]

progressively diminishes. The mice develop a 95% incidence of bilateral complex tubular adenomas of the ovary by 5 months of age.

It is of interest that Andervont and Dunn[8] found nine GCT among 98 tumors they saw in 225 wild house mice—seven in 99 autopsied breeding females, and two in 72 autopsied virgin females.

Rat

Ovarian neoplasms occur with some frequency in certain strains of rat. Katherine Snell[184] reported the incidence of tumors of various kinds in six inbred strains of rat in the laboratory of Pathology of the National Cancer Institute in Bethesda, Maryland (ACI, BUF, F344, OM, M520 and WN). GCT were found in about one-third of the OM rats over 18 months of age, only a few being found in ACI, M520 and, WN rats and none in BUF and F344. A few OM rats had simple papillary cystadenocarcinoma of the ovary. (Snell[184] refers to other reports of ovarian GCT, fibromas, adenomas, sarcomas, and carcinomas in rats.)

Lingeman[123] stated that the Registry of Experimental Cancers of the National Cancer Institute lists epithelial neoplasms in the ovaries of five untreated rats; of these, four were papillary cystadenocarcinomas, two of which contained foci of chondrosarcoma and had given widespread implantation peritoneal metastases.

In a period of 15 years, three ovarian tumors (excluding lymphomas) were found[28] in about 300 female Chester Beatty stock rats, including one GCT, one cystadenoma, and one anaplastic sarcoma. One of the most interesting recorded ovarian neoplasms in rats[175] is the spontaneous hormone-producing metastasizing GCT discovered by Iglesias et al.[100,101] in a female A × C rat. Symeonidis and Mori-Chavez[193] found a transplantable papillary adenocarcinoma in a 9-month-old OM rat. Other authors have recorded GCT in rats, e.g., Kullander,[118] who saw two GCT, along with one mixed androblastoma and GCT and one androblastoma; Thompson and Hunt[198] (see for review of literature) found one GCT and one papillary adenocarcinoma. In view of the peculiar Sertoliform structure of some bovine and canine GCT, the report by Engle[57] of the occurrence of testislike tubules and tubular adenomas in the ovaries of aged Wistar rats (Figures 39.11, 39.12, and 39.13), shrew,[211] and other mammals[211] (for references see Weir[206]) are relevant, even if they have no human counterpart.[123]

Guinea pig

Although GCT may occur,[107] the most interesting ovarian tumor of the guinea pig is the teratoma.[92,205] Willis[212] described a teratoma measuring 2 cm in a 9-week-old guinea pig and another 8.5 by 5.5 by 3 cm in a 1-year-old animal. Vink[203] also saw two ovarian teratomas in approximately 13,000 autopsies. Mosinger[145] refers to ovarian embryoma and to chorioepitheliomatous-like nodules described by Loeb;[125] they have limited duration, being destroyed and replaced by fibrous tissue.

Hamster

Handler[91] referred in his review of spontaneous lesions in Syrian hamsters to reports by Fortner[69] and by Kirkman of thecoma of the ovary.

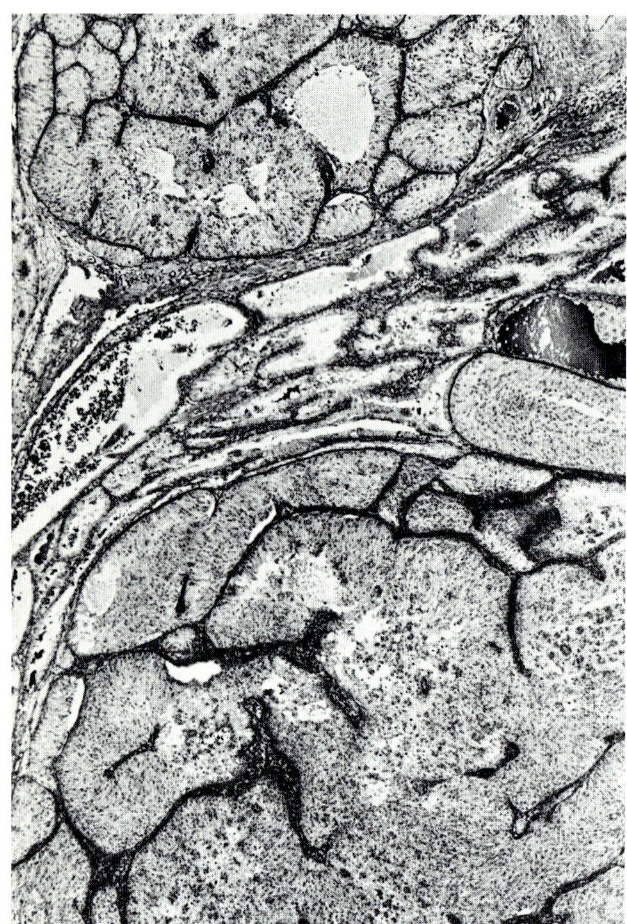

39.12 Tubular adenoma of the ovary of a rat. ×32.
[From a section kindly provided by D. S. G. Patton.]

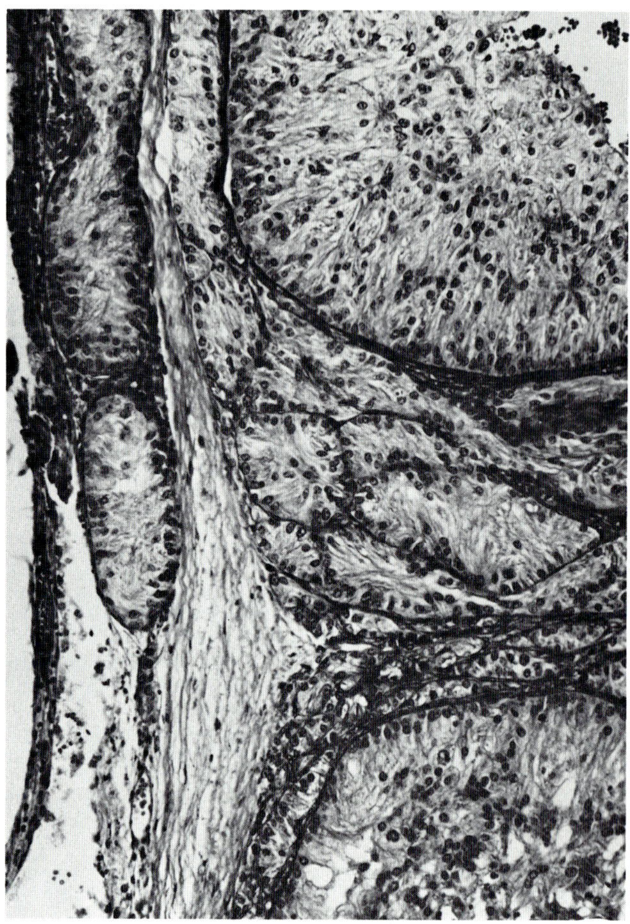

39.13 Same tumor as Figure 39.12, showing Sertoliform morphology. ×127.
[From a section kindly provided by D. S. G. Patton.]

Gerbil

Rowe et al.[173] found GCT in three of their gerbils; one also had a uterine leiomyosarcoma and showed bilateral symmetrical alopecia. The other two also had endometrial adenocarcinoma. One *M. shawi* had a bilateral granulosa–theca cell ovarian tumor as well as a unilateral ovarian papillary cystadenoma. Two gerbils, *M. shawi* and *G. hesperinus,* had leiomyomas of the ovary.

Ferret

In a stock of 123 female ferrets over 1 year of age, Chesterman and Pomerance[30] found bilateral ovarian thecomas; the endometrium had marked glandular hyperplasia. They also reported bilateral ovarian fibromyomas in a ferret, aged 5 years 4 months, which had been on a hepatotoxic diet for a short time about 4 years before its death.

Mastomys

Lingeman[123] reported a personal communication from Katherine Snell that malignant granulosa cell tumors are frequent in mastomys [*Praomys* (*Mastomys*) *natalensis*].

Wild Animals, Animals in Zoos, and Birds

Goyon[78] found a metastasizing teratoma in the left ovary of a hare, and Lombard[128] diagnosed a peculiar lesion in the ovary of a young hare as a seminoma. Flux[68] records some interesting findings in the ovaries of female

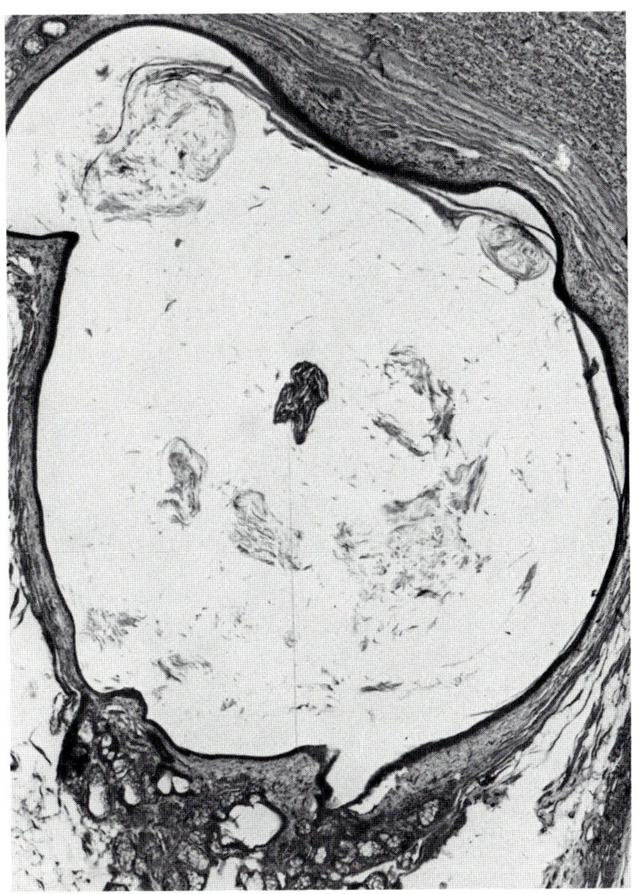

39.14 Teratoma of the ovary of a hare, showing cyst containing keratin and lined by stratified squamous epithelium, and groups of sebaceous glands (bottom). ×32. [From material kindly provided by Dr. J. E. Flux.]

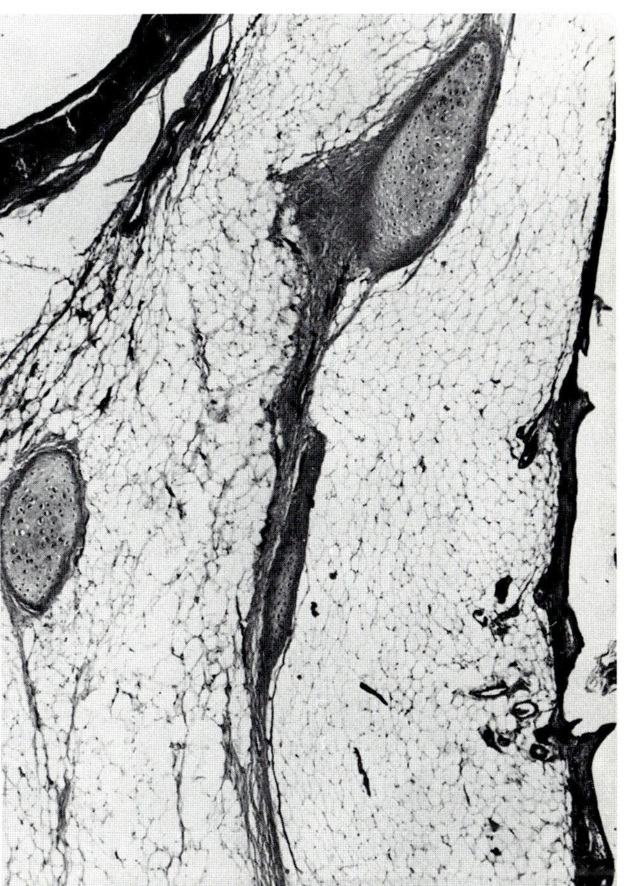

39.15 Teratoma of the ovary of a hare (same tumor as Figure 39.14), showing the wall of the epidermoid cyst (right), adipose tissue, and cartilage plates. ×32. [From material kindly provided by Dr. J. E. Flux.]

hares (*Lepus europaeus*) shot in New Zealand. Of 1,176 ovaries from adult hares, 48 contained cysts. Most of these cysts were filled with clear or opaque jelly or white, yellow, or green greasy sebaceous material. Six hares had true teratomas (Figures 39.14 through 39.18), containing teeth or bone (in four ovaries) and hair (in three). All six also had cysts filled with sebaceous material. The original liberation of hares in New Zealand in 1851 numbered only a few animals; the possibility is mentioned that a genetic susceptibility might be involved or an effect resulting from DDT spraying.

Dehner et al.[47] recorded a teratoma and a dysgerminoma in a ground squirrel, and Nowotny[155] a GCT in a squirrel (*Sciuris vulgaris* L.). In a chamois goat showing signs of masculinization, Dewalque[49] found a GCT of the left ovary which was surgically removed. Signs of masculinization reappeared 7 months later. The endometrium was hyperplastic and a histologic metastasis was found in one uterine cornu. In a koala (*Phascolarctos cinereus*), an Australian marsupial, Finckh and Bolliger[65] found a serous cystadenoma which appeared to arise from ovarian surface epithelium. Weir[206] found bilateral ovarian papillomata in an agouti (a dasyproctid member of the rodent suborder Hystricomorpha). The left ovary of a southern elephant seal (*Mirounga leonina*) contained what was taken to be a malignant GCT.[136] In their small series of tumors from whales, Rewell and Willis[167] reported a mucinous cystadenoma of the ovary, about 12 inches across, in a blue whale (*Balaenoptera musculus*) and presumed GCT in a pregnant blue whale and in two fin whales (*B. physalus*), one of which was pregnant.

Halloran[90] lists references to the following tumors in

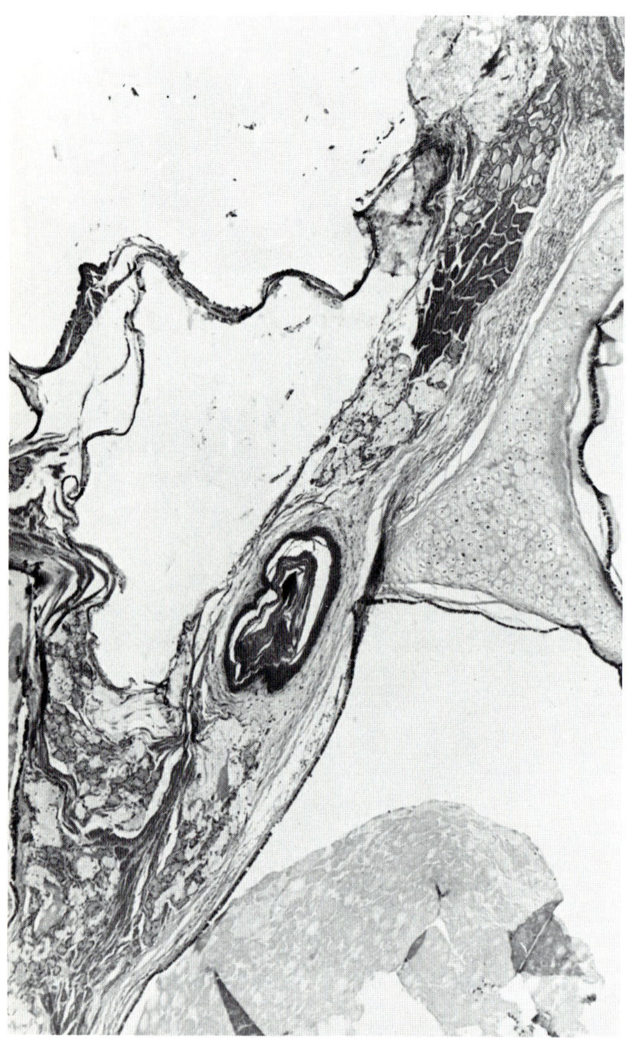

39.16 Teratoma of the ovary of a hare, showing cysts, salivary gland tissue (lower left), keratin (center), and cartilage (right). ×32.

[From material kindly provided by Dr. J. E. Flux.]

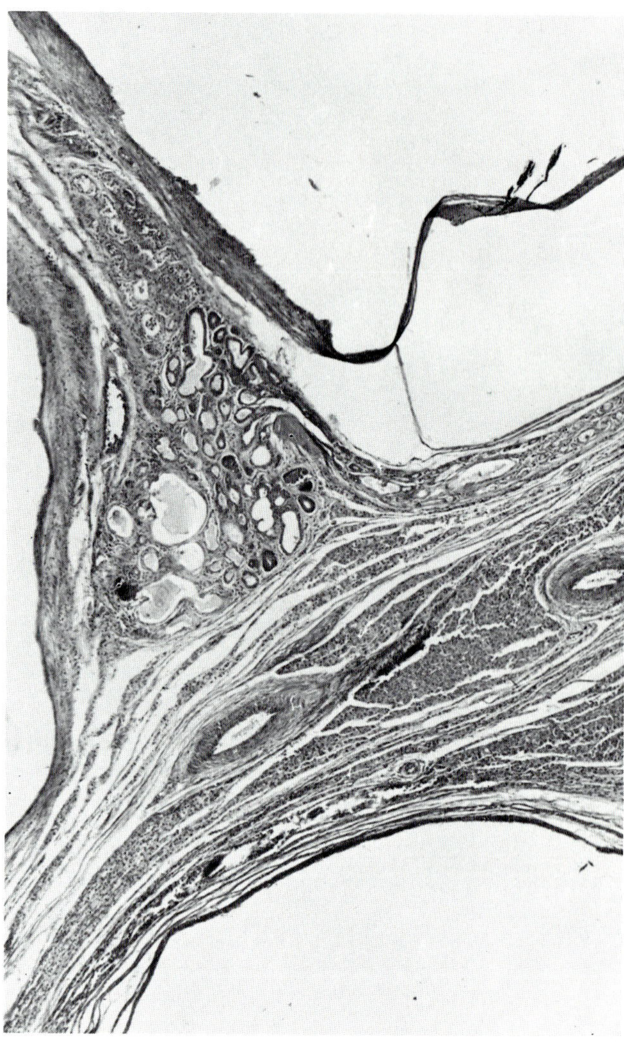

39.17 Teratoma of the ovary of a hare, showing cysts and glandular tissue. ×32.

[From material kindly provided by Dr. J. E. Flux.]

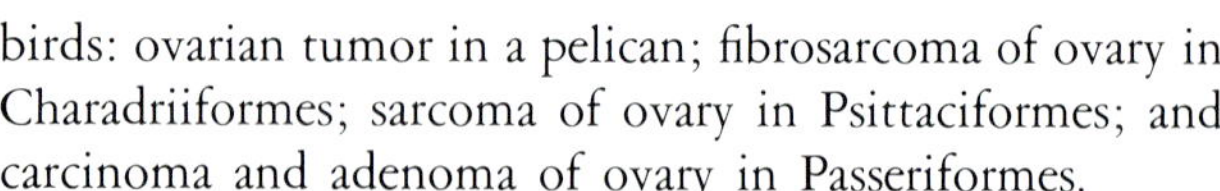

birds: ovarian tumor in a pelican; fibrosarcoma of ovary in Charadriiformes; sarcoma of ovary in Psittaciformes; and carcinoma and adenoma of ovary in Passeriformes.

Streett,[188] dissecting an adult female *Rana pipiens*, found a teratoma in the posterior pole of the right ovary, measuring 12 by 8 by 8 mm. Representative tissues of all three germ layers were present, including cartilage, bone, bone marrow, gut, and skin. A tumor in a *R. pipiens*, which was illustrated by Abrams,[2] was considered to be an ovarian cystadenocarcinoma (the kidney, the common site of tumors in this species, was free of tumor). According to Balls and Clothier,[15] Plehn in 1906 reported an ovarian carcinoma in *R. esculenta*.

In a survey of 44 avian and 11 mammalian cases of neoplasia in free-living wild mammals and birds in Britain, Jennings[108] found the following ovarian tumors: dysgerminoma in a mallard (*Anas platyrhynchos*), GCT also in a mallard, cystadenoma in a black-headed gull (*Larus ridibundus*), and arrhenoblastoma in a pheasant (*Phasianus colchicus*).

West[208] found a gonadal tumor, with an epithelial tubular structure, in the position of the ovary in a chukar

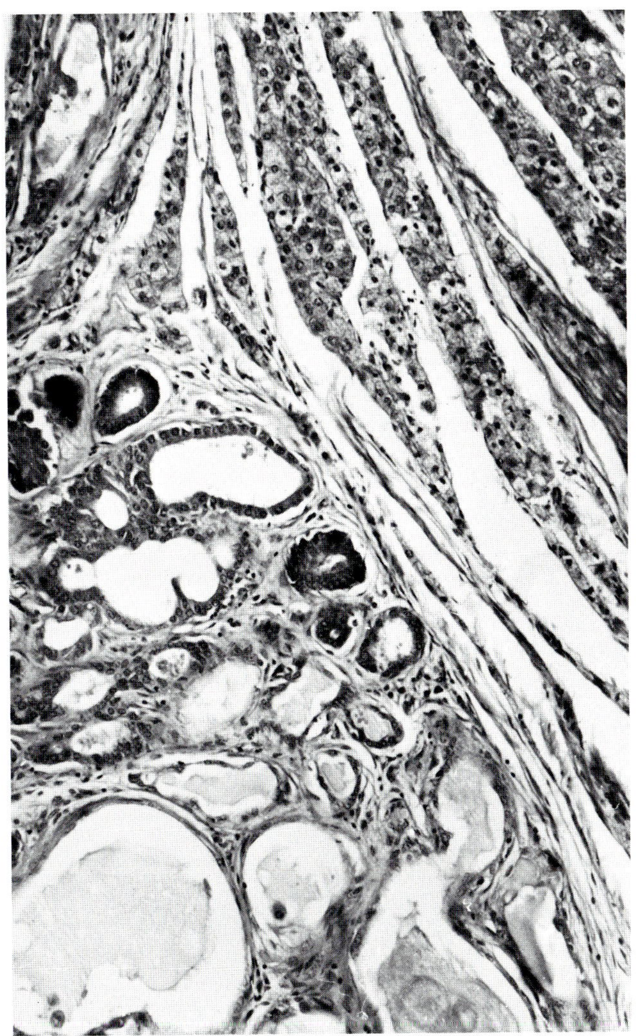

39.18 Teratoma of the ovary of a hare (same tumor as Figure 39.17), showing glandular tissue. ×127. [From material kindly provided by Dr. J. E. Flux.]

partridge from a game farm. The bird was typically female in appearance. The oviduct was present but incompletely mature.

Insect Study

Mention may be made of ovarian lesions in *Drosophila melanogaster.* King[114] states that "Two recessive mutations that render homozygous females sterile, because ovarian tumors are produced, have been extensively studied. The tumorous chambers seen in the ovaries of homozygotes contain cells resembling germarial cystocytes. Such chambers grow slowly by mitosis and some eventually contain as many as 10,000 cells. Cell division continues when tumors are transplanted to new hosts. However, the tumors do not invade nonovarian tissues and apparently have little effect on the viability of the donor or the host" (p. 325).

Domesticated Animals with Most Frequently Reported Tumors

Most information about ovarian tumors in domesticated animals refers to the mare, cow, cat, fowl, and bitch, and these species are now considered.

Mare

Ovarian tumors are not very rare in horses. Most of them are GCT (Figures 39.19 through 39.22) and most occur in young adults (see Finocchio and Johnson[66] for colored photographs, Mastronardi and Potena[135] for photomicrographs, and Burghardt[24] for ovarian cysts). It is uncertain what type of tumor affected the ovary of a foal reported by Christl[32] as no histologic support for the macroscopic diagnosis of cystadenoma was given. Among the reports of GCT are those by Howard,[99] Wurster,[215] and Leopold[120] (who also reviewed previous cases of GCT in mares and cows) and by Fessler and Brobst.[64] In the Fessler and Brobst case, the neoplastic left ovary, weighing over 1 kg, was removed from a 9-year-old mare that was infertile, showed anestrus, and developed malelike appearance and behavior. These signs regressed after the operation.

Teratomas appear to affect the ovary less frequently than the testis in the horse. Abraham[1] found the right ovary of a 10-year-old Quarter Horse mare to contain a tumor, approximately 12 by 10 by 10 cm, with cystic spaces lined by stratified squamous epithelium and filled with hair. The mare was multiparous but had failed to breed at three successive cycles. A teratoma in the right ovary of a 6-year-old Percheron mare[70] was located as a projection in a unilocular pseudomucinous cystadenoma.

The key papers on ovarian tumors in mares are those by Norris et al.[153] and by Cordes.[36] It is of interest that in the series of GCT in six horses and one Peruvian wild ass reported by the former, none were known to cause endocrine abnormality. The affected animals ranged from 4 to 31 years of age, and the tumors weighed 1 to 8 kg. They were yellowish, usually multicystic masses, with focal ne-

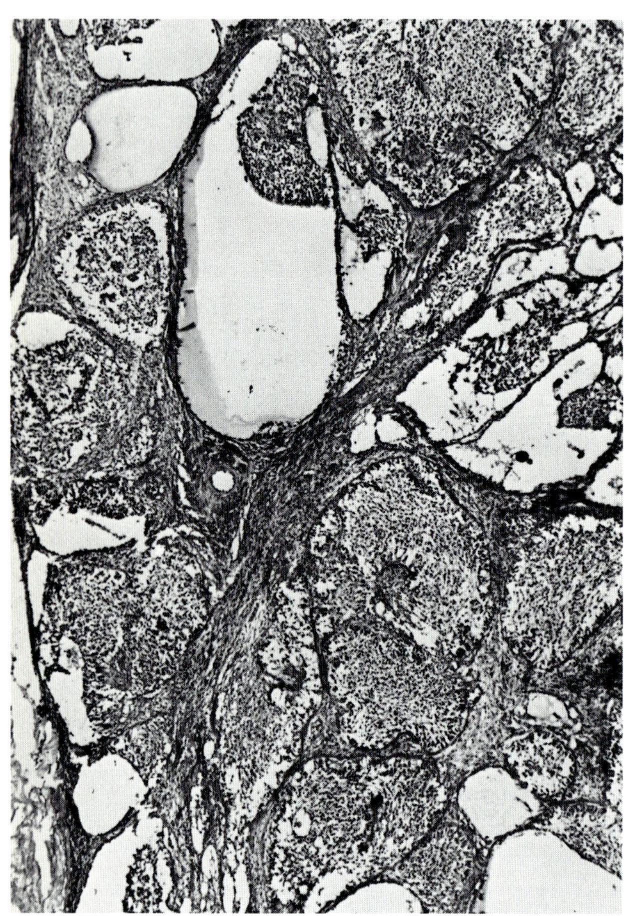

39.19 GCT of the ovary of a 13-year-old mare, showing tubular pattern. ×32.

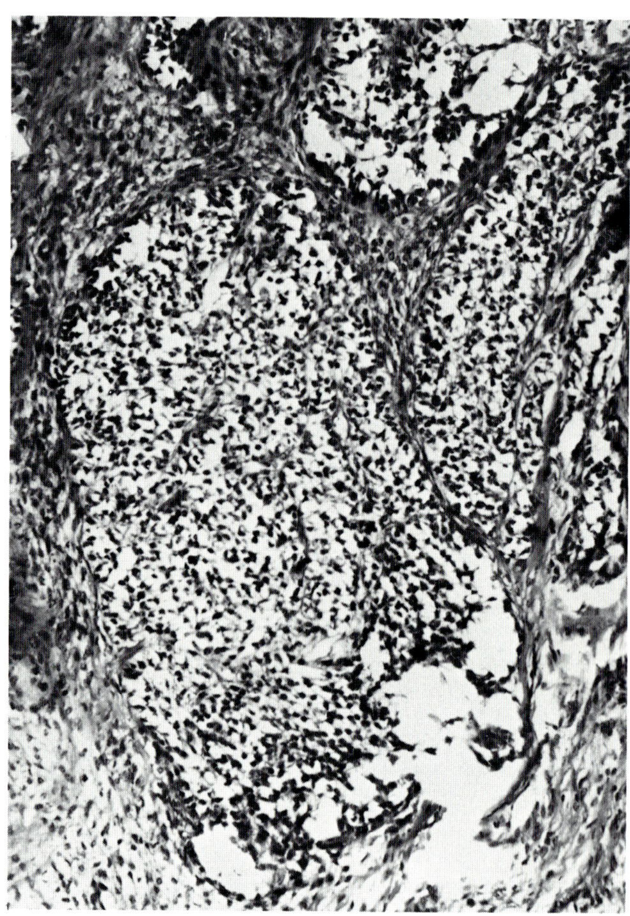

39.20 Same tumor as Figure 39.19. ×127.

crosis and hemorrhage. Histologically, the tumors showed prominent microcysts and tubules, with cells at the periphery of the cysts in double-paired layers, with basally oriented nuclei. These cells resembled the cells at the periphery of developing follicles and the Sertoli cells of the testis. A prominent stroma of spindle cells, possibly representing a thecal component, was present in all the tumors.

Cordes[36] studied nine cases of GCT in mares. All the tumors were removed surgically, eight from racehorse mares and one from a pony mare. The age (known for five mares) ranged from 7 to 16 years. Three tumors affected the right ovary and four the left. They were in mares with prolonged estrus (in one case there were clinical signs of masculinization) and were detected by rectal palpation. One grew from approximately 7 to 23 cm in 10 months. Eight were multicystic, the largest cyst being 3 cm in diameter. The tumor cells were chiefly in a follicular pattern, and theca cells were prominent. Some of these mares had given birth to foals prior to the neoplasms being detected, and they usually returned to normal after an operation.

Cow

The incidence of ovarian neoplasms in cows has been variously estimated. Although Davis, Leeper, and Shelton,[46] in their Denver abattoir survey, reported that five of the six ovarian tumors they recorded in cows were carcinomas (the sixth was diagnosed as a hypernephroma), the commonest form seems to be the GCT, of which Lagerlöf and Boyd[119] found 13 examples (including three carcinomas and three GCT) in the examination of 6,286 bovine genital tracts. Brandly and Migaki[21] found 13 GCT in 1,000 chronologically received tumors from veter-

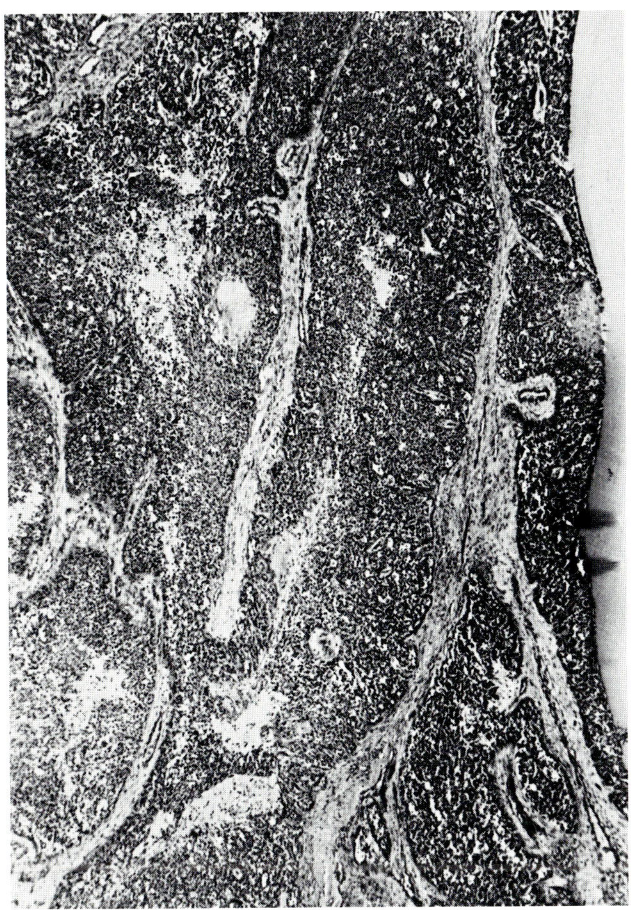

39.21 GCT of the ovary of a 30-year-old pony mare, showing solid pattern. ×32.

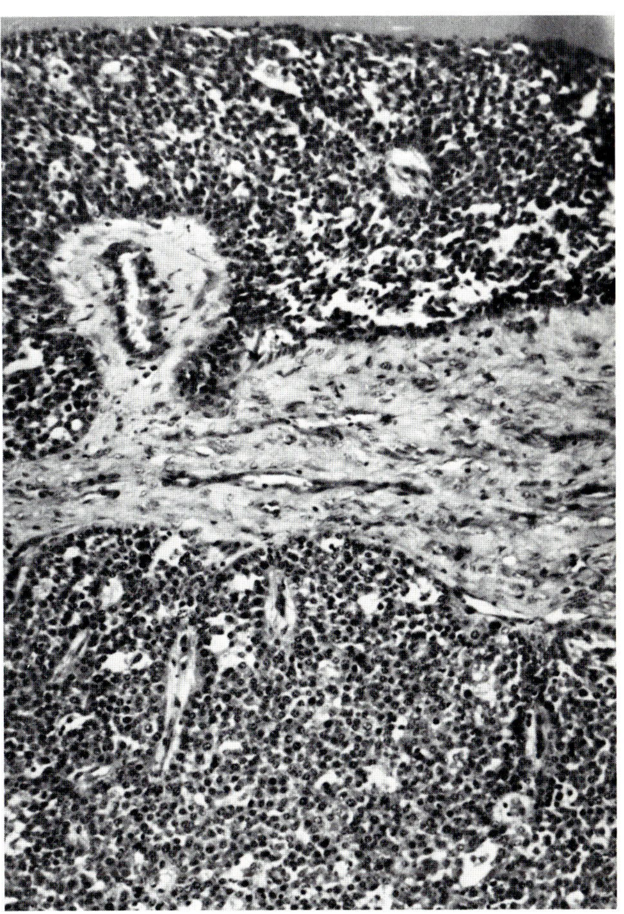

39.22 Same tumor as Figure 39.21. ×127.

inary meat inspectors. Anderson *et al.*,[7] in their British abattoir survey, found 302 tumors of all kinds from about 1.3 million cattle. There were 11 ovarian tumors—seven carcinomas (three serous cystadenocarcinomas, three mucinous adenocarcinomas,[191] one adenoacanthoma), two GCT, one combined teratoma–GCT, and one fibroma. In his abattoir survey in Holland, Misdorp[142] found 21 ovarian tumors in cows—10 GCT, seven carcinomas, and four thecomas.

The ages of affected cattle with GCT range from newborn[110] to 21 years[217] but the majority of tumors have been reported in animals of about 2 or 3 years of age. An interesting endocrinologic analysis was made by Short et al.[183] of a case of GCT in a Friesian heifer. At the age of 2 years 2 months, the heifer was noted to be showing enlargement of the udder. She developed certain behavior changes—mounting other animals in the herd but being seldom mounted herself. Her voice became more bull-like, and she pawed and horned the ground as a bull would. The tail head was found to be raised and the neck somewhat thickened, but the sacroiliac ligaments were not relaxed. When the heifer was sexually excited, an erectile structure, a fold of dorsal vaginal mucosa, appeared at the vulva. Lactation was noted. Rectal examination showed an enlarged left ovary and the heifer was destroyed. The ovarian tumor, approximately 15 cm in diameter, contained many cystic spaces and was a typical GCT, without luteinized cells. The endometrium showed signs of excessive progestational stimulation. The fluid in the tumor cysts contained progesterone, 20β-hydroxypregn-4-en-3-one, possibly a trace of 17α-hydroxyprogesterone, and estradiol-17β. It is suggested that the estradiol-17β came from normal theca interna cells, which surrounded some of the cystic follicles, or was being produced by neoplastic granulosa cells. The further comment is made that although the progesterone:estradiol-17β ratio was only 6:1, the tumor appeared to have caused normal mammary development and lactation.

Bovine GCT may be large tumors; the largest of Baumann's[17] five cases was 48 cm long and weighed 17.10 kg.

An important paper on bovine ovarian tumors is that by Norris, Taylor, and Garner,[154] who have studied the cases on file at the AFIP Registry of Veterinary Pathology. They classify the tumors as in the following tabulation.

Tumor type	No.
Ovarian stromal tumors	26
Granulosa type	13
Sertoli type	13
Teratoma	3
Carcinoma, primary site uncertain	3
Sarcoma, unclassified	2
Mixed mesodermal tumor	1
Metastatic lymphoma	1
Unclassified	3
Total	39

The main contribution these authors have made is to draw attention to the possible clinical significance of distinguishing typical GCT, composed of cells resembling typical granulosa cells, from what they term "Sertoli-type" ovarian stromal tumors; the former are much more prone to produce metastases.

Typical GCT occurred in animals 1.2 to 9 years of age (median 5 years). Two of the cows had nymphomania, and a third would not accept service by the bull. The tumors showed a consistent microfollicular pattern. Nine of the 13 cases of GCT of granulosa type showed metastases. The metastases occurred mainly to the broad ligament, to pelvic and abdominal peritoneal surfaces, and along the lumbar aorta. Two tumors had metastasized to the spleen and one to the lung. It was possible to examine the endometrium histologically in two cows: one showed a metastastic GCT and the other a pyometra.

The Sertoliform GCT arose in cows 4 to 12 years of age (median 8 years). Eleven were incidental findings. One cow had persistent pyometra, and one had shown an abdominal mass and estrus lasting 1 year. Hemorrhage and necrosis occurred in only three tumors, in contrast with the granulosa cell type. The tubular Sertolian arrangement was accompanied, in five tumors, by small areas of typical granulosa cell pattern. The authors describe and picture cells resembling Sertoli cells in the peripheral layer of early bovine granulosa follicles, prior to and during antrum formation.

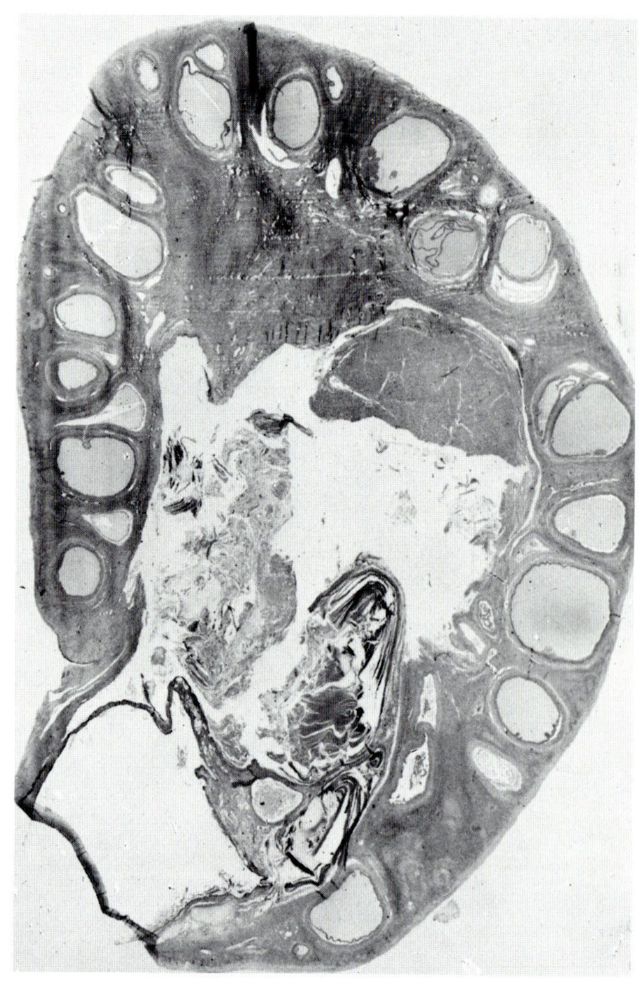

39.23 Teratoma of the ovary of a Zebu cow, showing keratin-filled cysts in depth of ovary (center lower left), and a superficial zone of Graafian follicles. Entire ovary.

[From material kindly provided by Dr. Silney A. Costa.]

Through the kindness of Dr. S. A. Costa, of Goiania, Brazil, I have been able to examine cases of peculiar cystic ovarian lesions he found in 13 of 4,008 slaughtered Zebu (Brahman) cattle. The lesions take the form of "dermoid cysts" and appear to be truly teratomatous in nature. The cysts, which vary in number from one to five in the sections I have studied, are rarely more than 2 cm across and are usually much smaller. They usually lie deep in the ovary (Figures 39.23 through 39.25) but in one instance

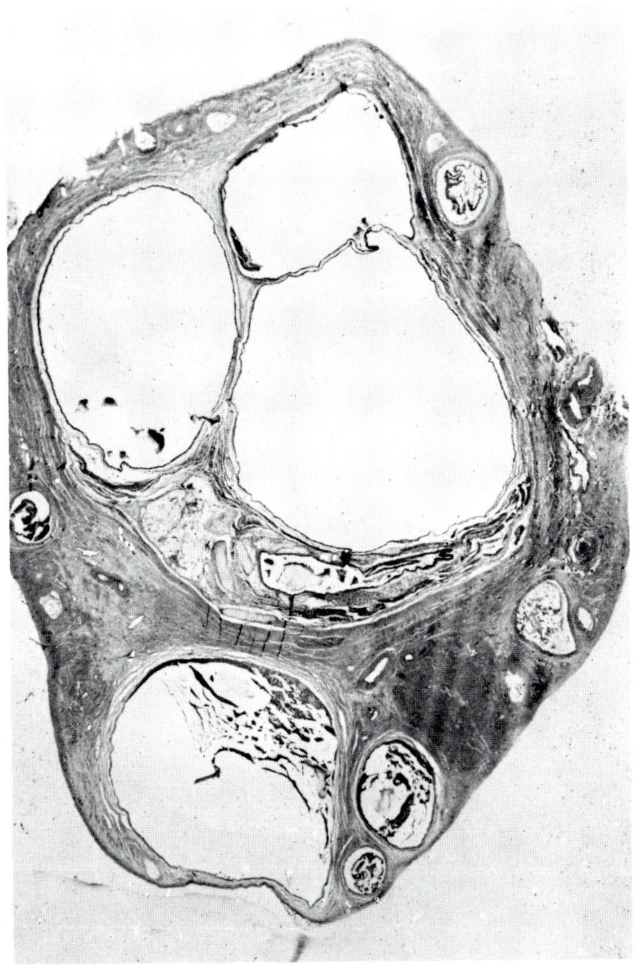

39.24 Teratoma of the ovary of a Zebu cow. There are four large deep cysts and, in the center, a focus of glands and cartilage. Entire ovary.

[From material kindly provided by Dr. Silney A. Costa.]

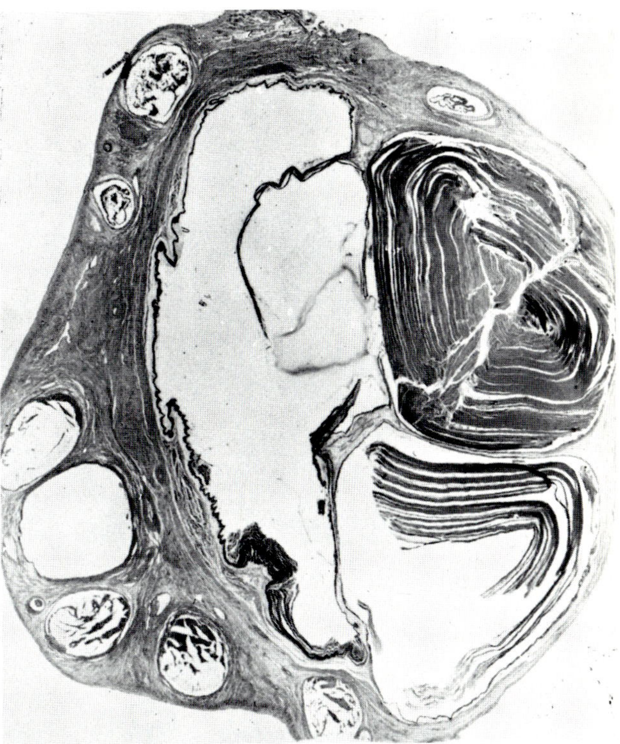

39.25 Teratoma of the ovary of a Zebu cow. There are four deep cysts, two filled with keratin.

[From material kindly provided by Dr. Silney A. Costa.]

the cyst is located no deeper than the Graafian follicles present. The cysts contain fluid or a colloid material or are more or less filled with keratinized squamous or dense keratin material. The typical cyst lining is stratified epithelium, from two to six or more cells thick, with keratin varying from scanty to massive. In one ovary there are patches of pseudostratified ciliated epithelium intermingled with the stratified epithelium, and in places goblet cells lie superficially on the stratified epithelium (Figure 39.26). In three ovaries the stratified epithelium is pigmented by melanin. In four ovaries from three cows, cartilage plates are present in the cyst walls (Figure 39.27). Three ovaries contain salivary glandlike tissue (Figure 39.27); one shows simple tubular glands; one has hair follicles, sebaceous, and sweat glands; one has sweat glands; and one has hair follicles. In two ovaries one and two neuronlike cells, respectively, are present.

The presence of hair follicles and of pigment allows these cysts to be called "dermoid" instead of "epidermoid." The presence of melanin and of salivary glandlike tissue and of possible neurons supports the diagnosis of teratoma. The histogenesis of the cysts is obscure. There is a hint in the superficial location of the cyst in one tumor, in the presence of keratin, squamous and possible squamous epithelium in the lining of a Graafian follicle in another, and the apparent continuity with structures resembling egg cords (or SES) in two sites in the wall of one cyst in a third (Figure 39.28) that they may originate from the Graafian follicles. Study of further such tumors may help decide the question.

Cat

Few ovarian tumors have been reported in cats, but in assessing the significance of this, the common practice of

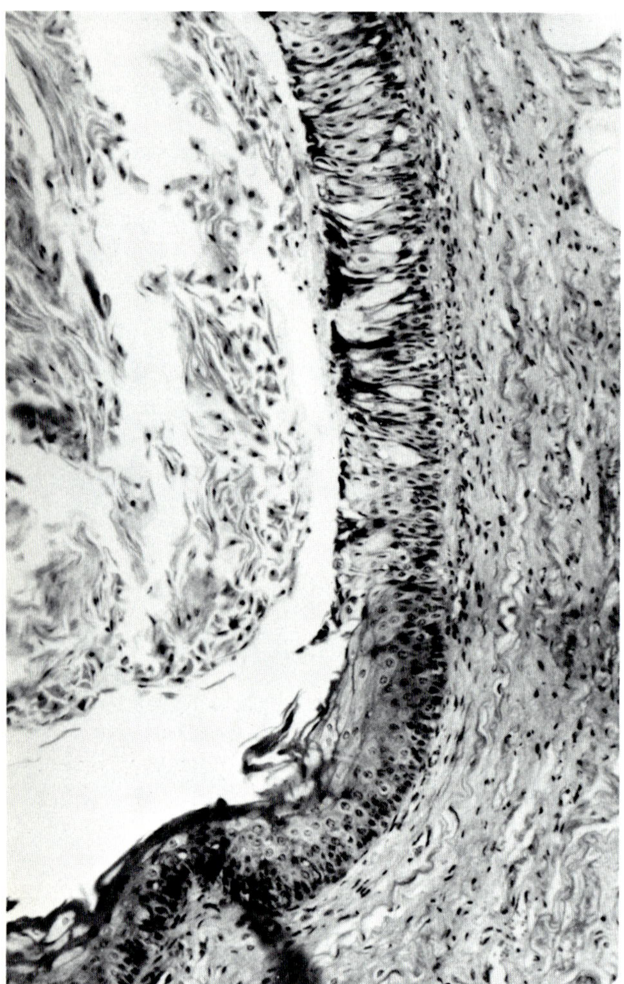

39.26 Teratoma of the ovary of a Zebu cow. Part of the wall of the cyst, showing stratified squamous and goblet cell epithelium merging. Same tumor as Figure 39.23. ×127.

[From material kindly provided by Dr. Silney A. Costa.]

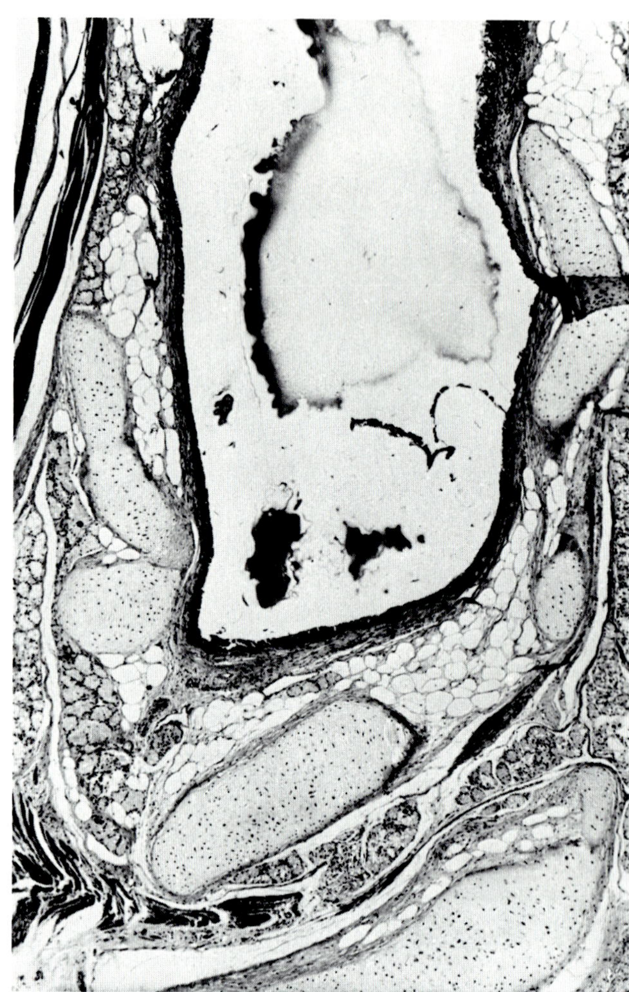

39.27 Teratoma of the ovary of a Zebu cow, showing cartilage plates in the wall of the cyst and salivary gland tissue. ×32.

[From material kindly provided by Dr. Silney A. Costa.]

spaying female cats must be remembered. The key paper is by Norris, Garner, and Taylor.[151] Other reports include those by Federer[59]; by Di Domizio[50] of GCT with lung and liver metastases; by Fukushima and Konishi[71] of GCT in a 3-year-old cat, with omental and kidney metastases; by Baker[14] of GCT; by Sbernardori and Nava[176] of dysgerminoma of the right ovary of a 7-year-old plurigravid cat; and by Dehner et al.[47] of two dysgerminomas (one metastasizing), one teratoma, and one mixed dysgerminoma and teratoma.

Norris et al.[151] studied 12 ovarian neoplasms from 10 cats and one lion (a leiomyoma). Six GCT were found in five cats of mixed domestic breed. All five cats showed signs of estrogen stimulation; two had prolonged estrus, thinning of coat, and loss of hair and three had endometrial hyperplasia. One cat also had a mammary carcinoma. Four tumors were unilateral. Three were 6 cm or more across, and three extended beyond the ovary. They were usually yellow cystic tumors with areas of hemorrhage, and were composed of small cells with hyperchromatic nuclei devoid of nuclear grooves; the arrangement was typically microfollicular and Call–Exner bodies were present in two tumors. Four neoplasms showed a minor theca cell component. A virilized 9-year-old cat had a lipid cell tumor;

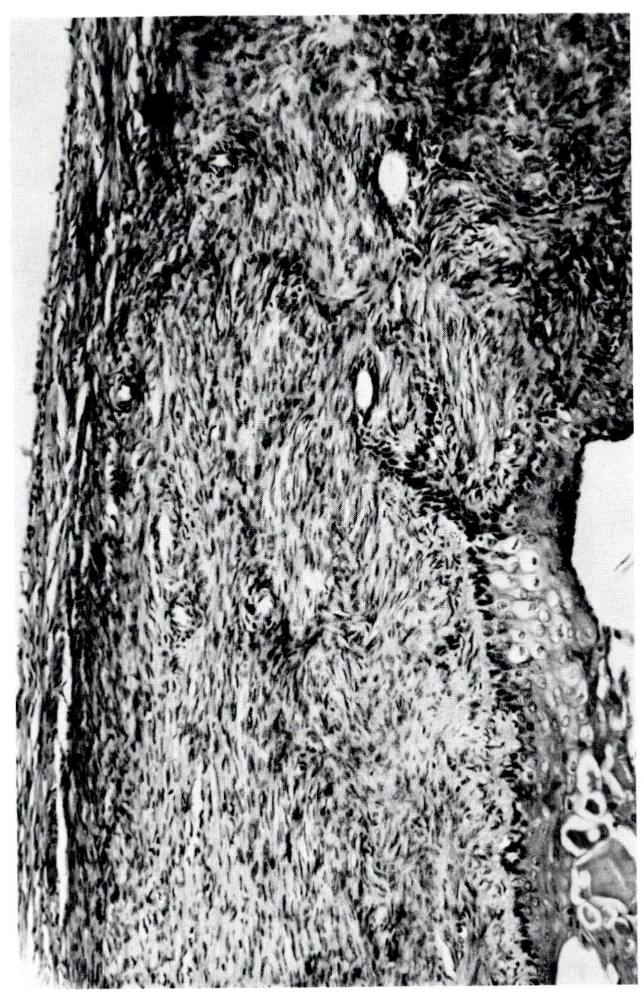

39.28 Teratoma of a Zebu ovary, showing apparent continuity of the epithelium lining the cyst and a subsurface epithelial structure. Surface of ovary on left. ×127.

[From material kindly provided by Dr. Silney A. Costa.]

the endometrium was cystic. There were two ovarian teratomas: The smaller had well-differentiated tissues, including cartilage, glial tissues, glandular epithelium, hair, keratin, and squamous epithelium, whereas the larger tumor had cells resembling those of human dysgerminoma in some areas. One tumor was a metastasizing adenocarcinoma, and the tenth cat, a 10-year-old Persian, showed metastasis of an endometrial carcinoma to both ovaries and elsewhere.

Norris et al.[151] comment on the absence of a Sertoliform pattern in feline GCT. They also state that ovarian capsular epithelium of the cat, unlike that of dog and man, shows little tendency toward hyperplasia with inclusion cyst formation.

Fowl

An extensive account of ovarian tumors in domestic fowl is given by Campbell,[26,27] which may be summarized as follows: Although formerly frequent, advanced adenocarcinoma of the hen's ovary is now comparatively rare because of the policy of discarding hens after their first or second year of reproductive life. Ovarian tumors of the granulosa–thecal–luteal type are not uncommon in broiler chickens aged 10 weeks or less. Ovarian adenocarcinomas are common in older hens and may have a high incidence in hens reared in a constant environment. The tumor, which may appear as a serous or mucous-secreting cystadenocarcinoma, may have an extensive plain muscle component and tends to form serosal implantation metastases.

Other tumors described by Campbell[26] include theca cell tumors, Brenner tumor, lipoid cell tumor, and hemangioma. Surgical removal of the left or functional ovary almost invariably leads to the development of an ovotestis in the right rudimentary ovary, from which tumors may later develop, including Sertoli cell adenoma or arrhenoblastoma and dysgerminoma.

Sparse reports of ovarian and oviductal tumors in Anatidae are reviewed by Rigdon,[169] who has observed a teratoma of the ovary region in two of 17 hermaphrodites which resulted from mating male Muscovy and female white Pekin ducks.

Dog

Types of canine ovarian tumors. The types of canine ovarian tumors encountered in four collections are summarized in Table 39.1.

The source of material in these reports varied. Dow's[55] material was collected at the Glasgow Veterinary School from histologically examined ovaries of 400 unselected autopsied bitches. Of these, 93 had a total of 127 tumors of various types in one or more sites. Twenty-five bitches (18 of which were nulliparous, ranging from 5 to 15 years of age) had primary ovarian tumors. One in 16 of the bitches therefore had an ovarian tumor. From the nature of the survey, no strong correlation with genital system symptoms would be expected. Dow's findings may be compared with those of Zaldivar.[219] In a series of Beagles in the Argonne colonies, he found spontaneous malignant tumors in 540 dogs: of these two were of ovarian origin

Table 39.1 Canine ovarian tumors in four collections

Tumor type	Investigator				Total
	Dow[a]	Cotchin[b]	Ishmael[c]	Norris et al.[d] and Dehner et al.[e]	
Group 1	11	25	14	33	83
Papilloma and Adenoma	10	20	8	20	
Carcinoma	1	5	6	3	
Intermediate				10	
Group 2	13	30	5	26	74
GCT	13	15	5	15	
Sertoliform		15		6	
Nonspecific				5	
Group 3	0	9	3	13	25
Seminoma		8	1	11	
Teratoma		1	2	2	
Group 4					14
Miscellaneous and undiagnosed	1	5	2	6	
Total	25	69	24	78	196

[a] Located in Glasgow; see Ref. 55.

[b] Located in London; see Ref. 39.

[c] Located in Liverpool; see Ref. 103.

[d] Located at Armed Forces Institute of Pathology, Washington, D.C.; see Ref. 152.

[e] Located at Armed Forces Institute of Pathology, Washington, D.C.; see Ref. 47.

(in 264 females), adenocarcinoma and granulosa cell carcinoma in 10-year-old animals. My own material[39] was a mixture of specimens obtained during surgery and at autopsy and therefore exaggerates the number of tumors coming from bitches with genital system symptoms. Ishmael's[103] series included material examined in the pathology laboratory of the Liverpool Veterinary School. The material reported by Norris et al.[152] (the dysgerminomas and teratomas being reported in detail by Dehner et al.[47]) was comprised of the 78 primary canine ovarian tumors on file in the Armed Forces Institute of Pathology Registry of Animal Pathology, again a selective collection.

The separation of tumors into different groups in Table 39.1 reflects my concept of their histogenesis. In Group 1 are included tumors of epithelial type, which develop from surface epithelium (papillomas) or from its extensions below the surface (adenomas). Some tumors are predominantly if not entirely papillomatous and there is often some adenomatous component. In Group 2 are included what Norris et al.[152] call gonadal stromal tumors but which are more commonly called by veterinary pathologists, especially in the United Kingdom, granulosa cell tumors. Group 3 includes tumors that morphologically resemble canine testicular seminomas, and teratomas. These are classed by Dehner et al.[47] as germ cell tumors. Group 4 includes miscellaneous tumors and tumors of uncertain type.

The following account of the various types of canine ovarian tumors is mainly based on my own report.[39]

Group 1: Papilloma and adenoma. The ages of 19 of my 20 bitches ranged from 4 to 15 years, with an average of 9.4 years (in Dow's series, the 10 animals were 6 to 13 years of age). In six of 13 bitches for which information was available, both ovaries were affected; the other tumors involved the left (five) or right (two) ovary alone. Six of the 20 bitches showed signs of hormonal disturbance ("pyometra" in four; cystic endometrial hyperplasia in two). Six other bitches showed signs of an enlarged abdominal mass.

Not unexpectedly, the tumors in Dow's autopsy series

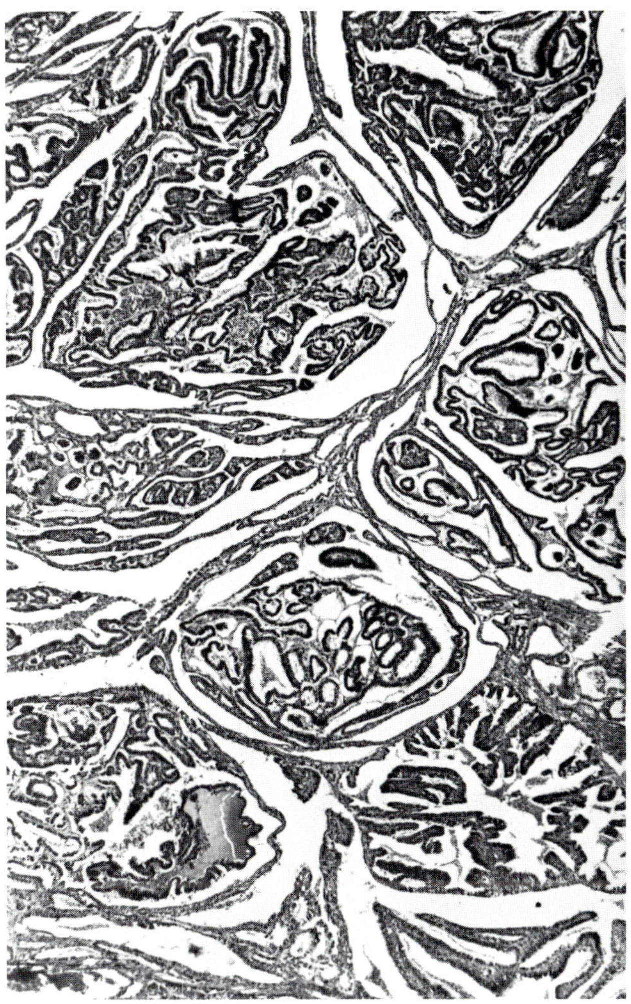

39.29 Adenoma of the ovary of a 9-year-old mongrel bitch. ×32.

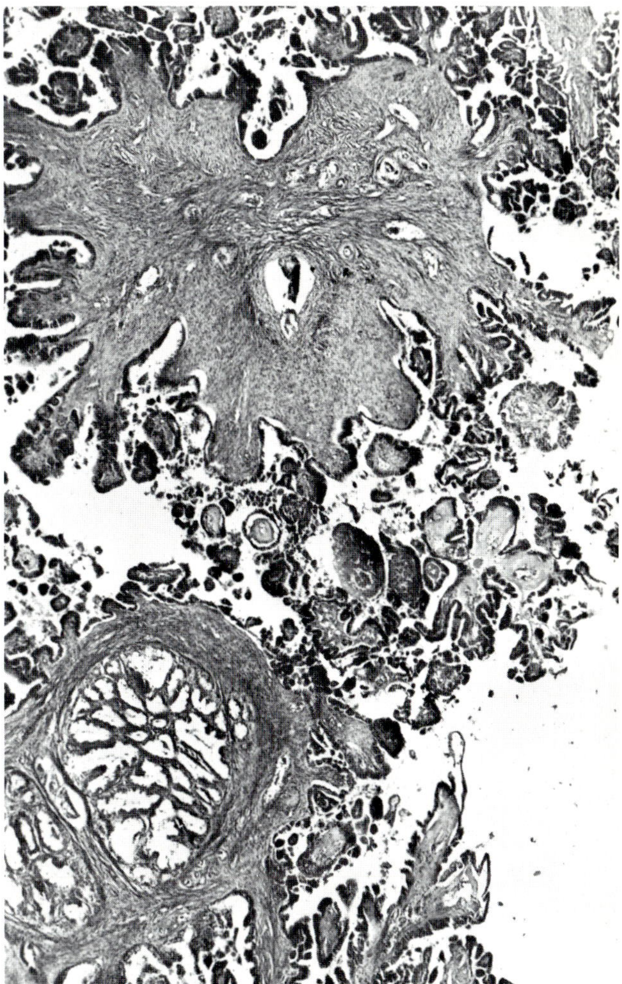

39.30 Papilloma and adenoma of the ovary of a 14-year-old crossbred bitch. ×32.

were generally small, ranging from 0.8 to 1.5 cm in diameter, although four of them (including two pseudomucinous cystadenomas) were from 6 to 10 cm diameter. In my series, one adenoma was a histologic finding in a bitch with a vaginal fibroma, the other tumors ranging from 1.5 to 17 cm in length (average 7 cm).

The macroscopic appearance of the tumors varied according to whether surface papilloma formation was present (five out of 20 dogs) or not. In at least six dogs, and probably in more, the tumor lay in an intact but distended bursa. The surface (apart from papillomatous tumors, which had a fine coxcomblike surface) was smooth but nodular or bosselated, and variably gray, yellowish, or hemorrhagic. The cut surface was partly solid and partly cystic. The solid areas were mostly grayish or pinkish white, and usually finely lobulated or papillary. The cysts varied in size and contained clear watery fluid, sometimes brown or bloodstained.

The histologic structure was predominantly that of a papillary cystadenoma (Figure 39.29) (cf. Fedrigo[60]) with a variable superficial papillary component (Figure 39.30). The cyst contents were hyaline. They were lined by one or sometimes more layers of cuboidal or columnar cells with basal or central nuclei; the papillae were supported by a connective tissue stroma, varying from fine to edematous, hyaline (Figure 39.31), and hemorrhagic. In five tumors, the prominent superficial papillomatous growths appeared in places to be continuous with the surface epithelium. In

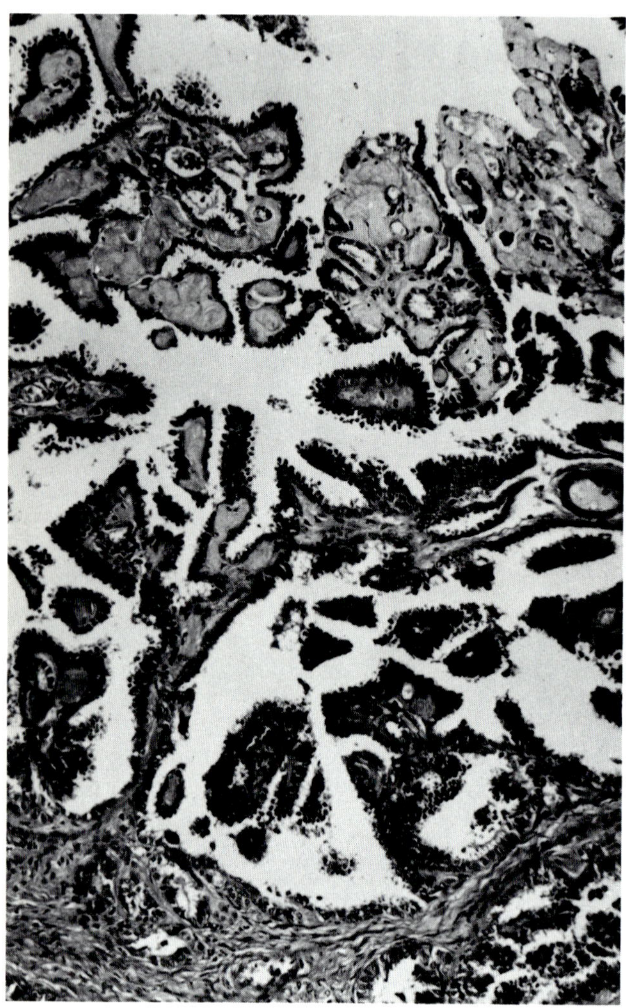

39.31 Papilloma of the ovary of a 10-year-old Alsatian bitch, showing hyalin cores of papillae. ×32.

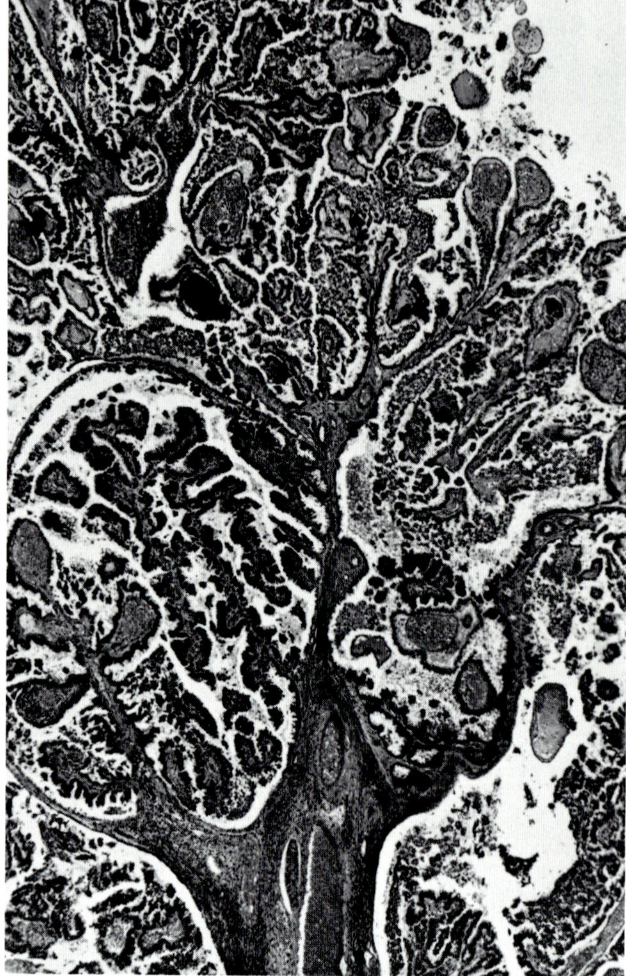

39.32 Papillary carcinoma of the ovary of a 15-year-old bitch. ×32.

six tumors, there were areas resembling GCT. Two of Dow's 10 cases were of the pseudomucinous type.

A sufficiently detailed histochemical analysis has not been made of my series, but the main if not the only type appears to be the serous cystadenoma.

Carcinoma. Carcinomas are less common in the bitch ovary than are adenomas. Dow has found one metastasizing carcinoma as against 10 adenomas; in my series, there have been five against 20; in the Norris et al.[152] series, even if the 10 intermediate tumors are classed as carcinomas, they form in total 13 against 20 adenomas. In my series, the average age of the affected dogs (9.5 years) was the same as for the bitches with ovarian adenoma (9.4 years). Four of the five bitches showed signs of hormonal disturbance ("pyometra," two; cystic endometrial hyperplasia, one; vaginal hemorrhage, one).

The tumors, from 3 to 10 cm long, showed a smooth, nodular surface, covering a homogenous or finely cystic whitish or yellowish tissue. They were histologically predominantly intracystic papillary tumors (Figure 39.32) with areas of compressed tubular structures and of anaplasia (Figure 39.33). Mitoses were present and lymphatic permeation was noted. Two of the affected bitches showed metastases; in both, the greater omentum was involved and fluid was present in excess in the abdomen. One of the bitches also showed, in addition to implantation metastases, lymph nodal and pulmonary deposits.

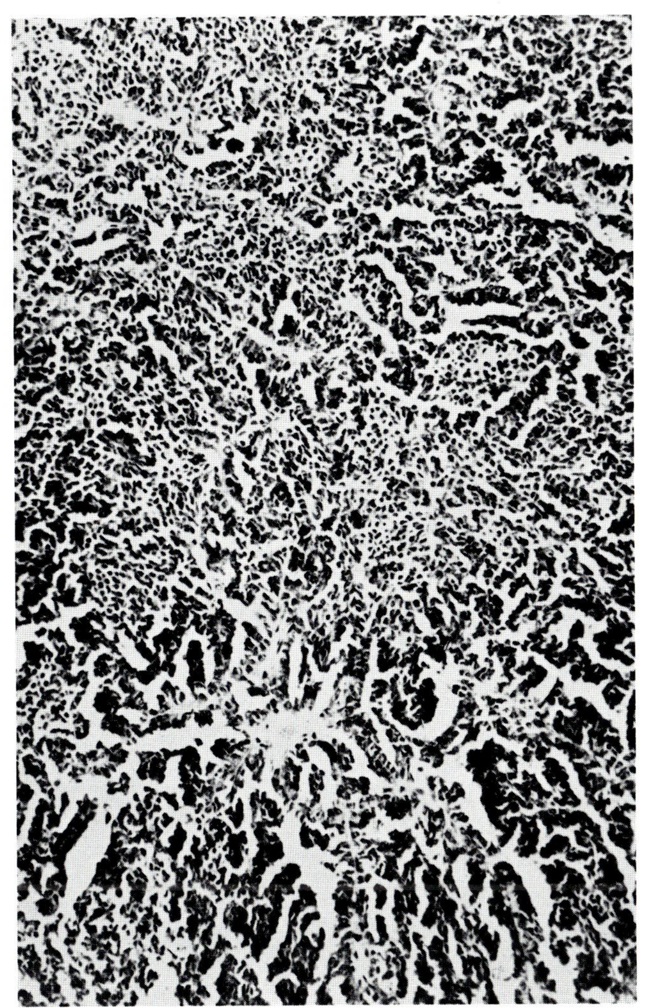

39.33 Anaplastic adenocarcinoma of the ovary of a 7-year-old hound-type bitch. ×127.

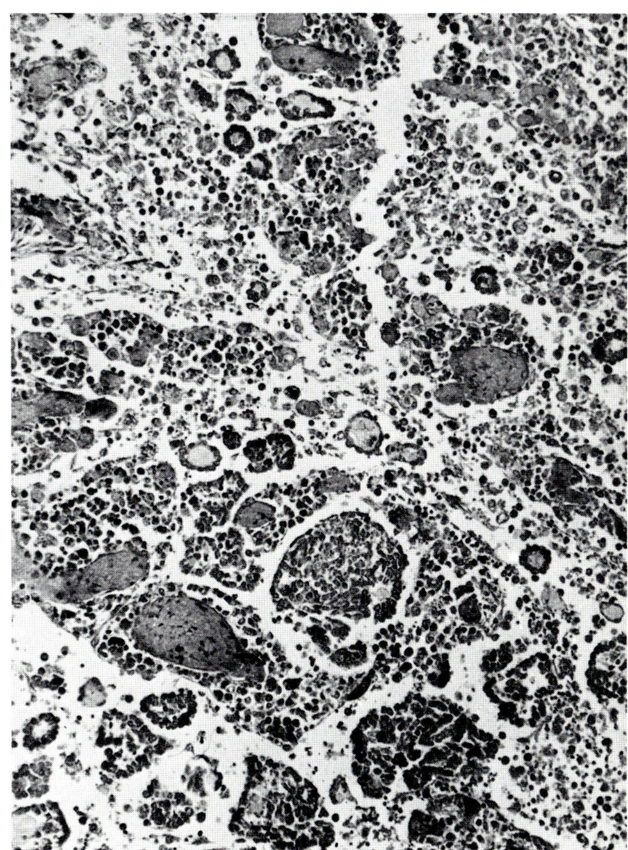

39.34 Nodal deposit, with globular epithelial formations, from an ovarian adenocarcinoma in a 9-year-old Terrier bitch. ×127.

Fedrigo and Rugiati[61] described the use of Papanicolaou smears to identify tumor cells in the ascitic fluid of a 4-year-old Alsatian bitch with a recurrent papillary adenocarcinoma of the right ovary. Chromosomal abnormalities (number and morphology) were demonstrated in the tumor cells. Addis and Baglioni[3] found apparent neoplastic elements in rosettes in May–Grunwald–Giemsa smears of recurrent ascitic fluid in a 6-year-old Alsatian bitch with an ovarian papillary "cystoadenoma" (sic). I have seen similar globes of tumor cells in a nodal deposit of a bitch with adenocarcinoma (Figure 39.34), and Case and Small[29] also illustrate such structures in the right iliac node of a 1½-year-old English Setter bitch with adenocarcinoma of the right ovary. In view of the presence of eosinophils in some ovarian tumors, it is of interest that Cork[37] found an elevated blood eosinophilia (up to 4.5%) in an 8-year-old mixed-breed bitch with a cystadenocarcinoma of the right ovary.

Group 2: Granulosa cell tumor (*GCT*). In their account of gonadal stromal tumors, Norris et al.[152] have separated (not solely on morphologic grounds) from the classic GCT a group that they call Sertoli pattern tumors (for which I use the adjective, Sertoliform) and another of nonspecific type. It appears possible that these are in fact all of granulosa cell or related origin. In my own series of 30 tumors classified as GCT, at least 15 had some more or less pronounced histologic resemblance to the canine Sertoli cell tumor (SCT).

The age range in my series of dogs with GCT (including Sertoliform tumors) was 1½ to 12 years, average 8.0. The Norris et al.[152] "granulosa" (non-Sertoliform) tumors

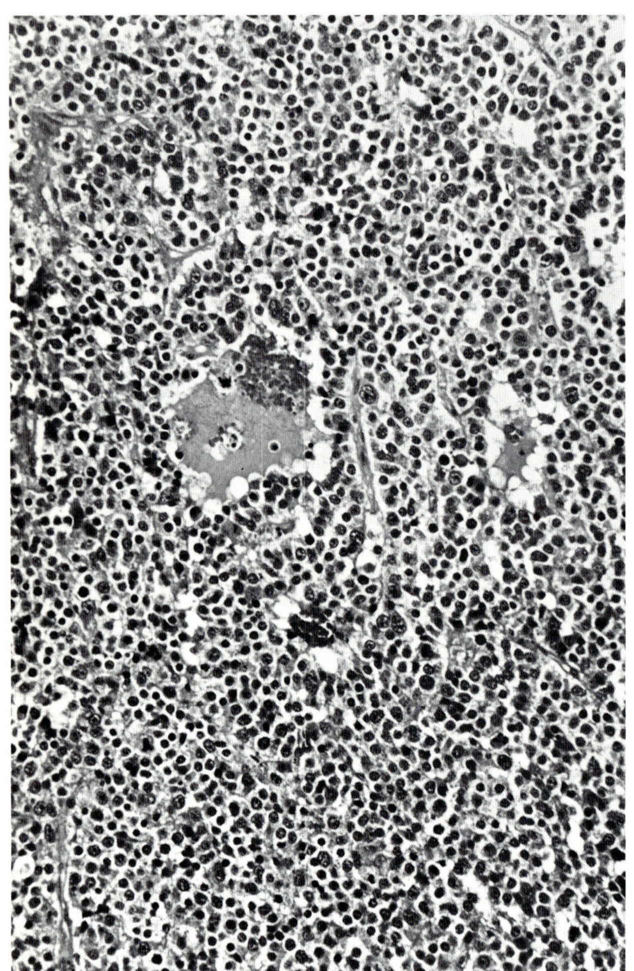

39.35 GCT of the ovary of an 11-year-old Labrador bitch, showing sheets of cells, follicular fluid pools, and fine connective tissue septa. ×127.

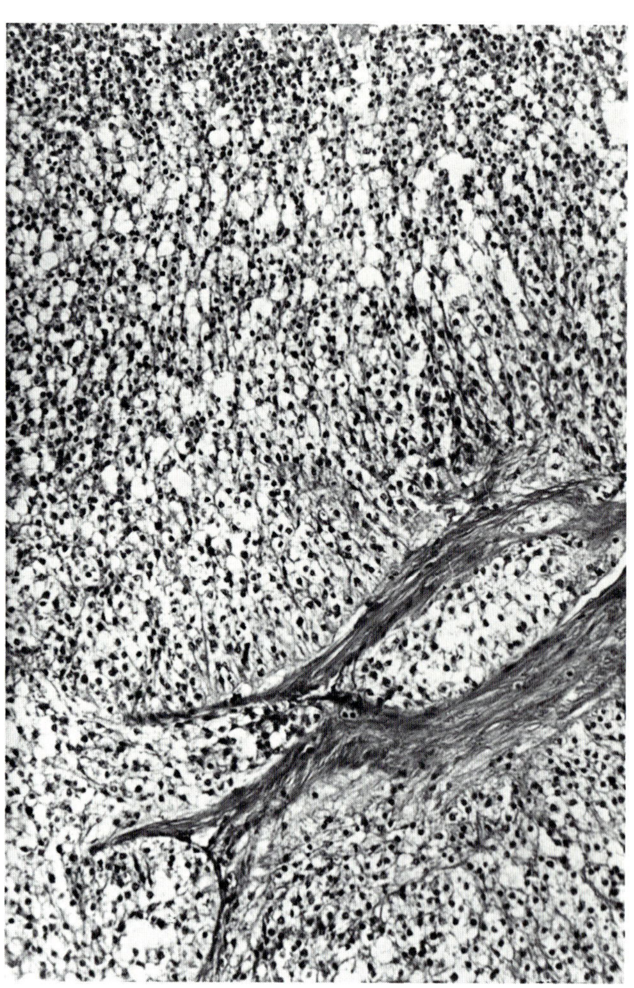

39.36 GCT of the ovary of a 5-year-old Alsatian bitch, showing coarse and fine stromal septa. ×127.

were found in bitches 4 to 12 years of age (median 7 years) but their six Sertoliform tumors were in dogs from 10 to 15 years of age (median 12 years). In both series, there is an indication of a tendency for Bulldogs and Boxers to be affected more often than other breeds. Twenty-three of my series of 30 bitches showed signs of hormonal disturbance: 19 had "pyometra," three had cystic endometrial hyperplasia, and one, which had shown no true estrus for 2 years, had remained persistently attractive to male dogs.

The tumors were large, varying from 5 to 11 cm in length with an average of 7 cm. They lay wholly or partly in a distended ovarian bursa. The surface was smooth, nodular, or bossellated and the color was gray or blue (from hemorrhage). The cut surface was partly solid and partly cystic, commonly with areas of hemorrhage.

Two of my cases showed metastases, one mainly as retroperitoneal extension and the other to nodes and viscera, including lung. Three of the Norris et al[152] "granulosa" tumors had local extension or metastasis; none of their six Sertoliform tumors had metastasized or extended locally beyond the ovary.

Histologically, the usual pattern was of connective tissue septa of varying thickness, usually broad, dividing the tumor cells into large groups (Figures 39.35 and 39.36) that were in turn divided into smaller groups by finer connective tissue septa. The tumor cells resembled either mature granulosa cells with rounded nuclei and eosinophilic or sometimes foamy, clear, or granular cytoplasm, sometimes arranged in a tubular pattern (Figure 39.37) or were more elongated and arranged in a Sertoli-

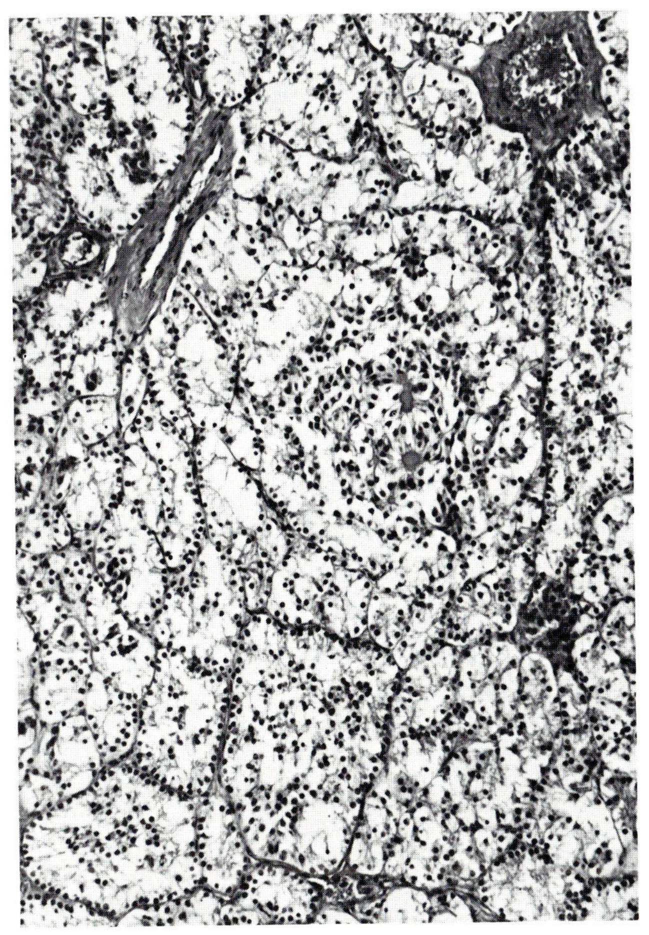

39.37 GCT of the ovary of a 10-year-old Retriever bitch, showing clear cells in tubular arrangement. ×127.

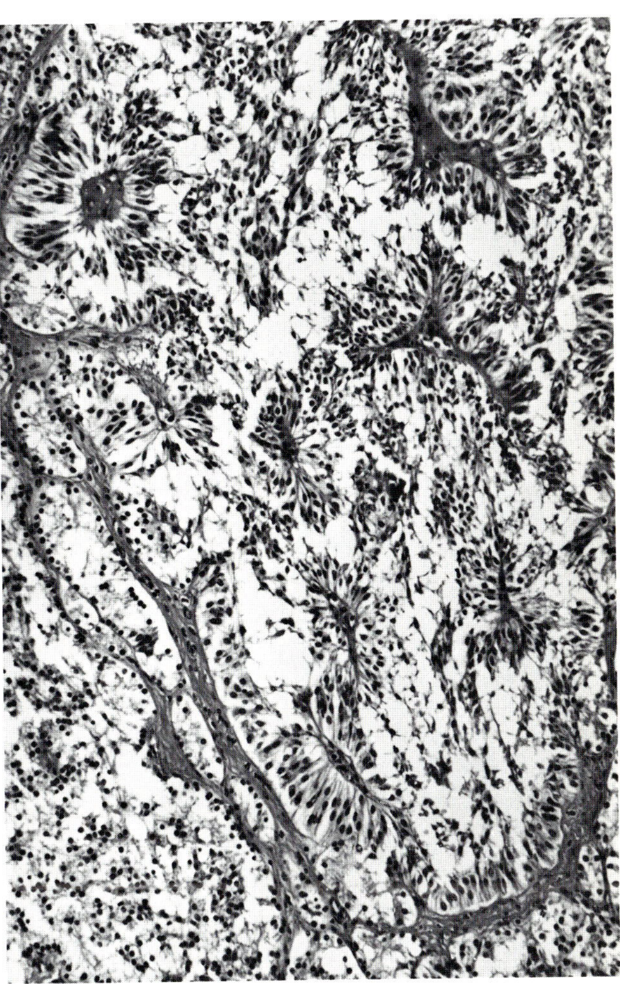

39.38 Sertoliform GCT of the ovary of a bitch (same tumor as Figure 39.37). ×127.

form fashion (Figures 39.38 and 39.39) Mitoses were sometimes readily found in the typical granulosa cell regions but were not readily found in Sertoliform areas. The presence of Call–Exner-like bodies (Figure 39.40) was not constant, but they were found in three of my cases. In some tumors, a marked perithelial arrangement was seen. Pools or lakes of hyaline material resembling follicular fluid were typically present.

There was a clear suggestion, in a least five tumors, that the granulosa-cell pattern was mixing (Figure 39.41) smoothly with a papillary or tubular adenoma, and a transition between typical granulosa cell and typical Sertoliform areas was also noted in some tumors.

Group 3: Seminoma (dysgerminoma). I have reported eight cases of a seminoma-like tumor of the canine ovary, Dehner et al.[47] have found 11, and Andrews et al.[9] have found two. The tumors bear a close histologic resemblance to canine testicular seminoma (see Buergelt[23]). It would be desirable that electron microscopic examinations be made to see whether this similarity exists at the ultrastructural level.

The bitches in my series ranged from 6 to 16 years of age, with an average of 10.5, which is a little above the average age for other forms of ovarian tumors. In this group, the dogs studied by Dehner et al.[47] were, on the average, considerably older (13 years) than their dogs[152] with GCT (7 years) and a little older than their dogs with Sertoliform tumors. Indeed Taylor and Dorn[194] saw a dysgerminoma in a 20-year-old Alsatian bitch. Signs of hormonal disturbance accompanied at least four of my eight seminomas—"pyometra" in two bitches, cystic en-

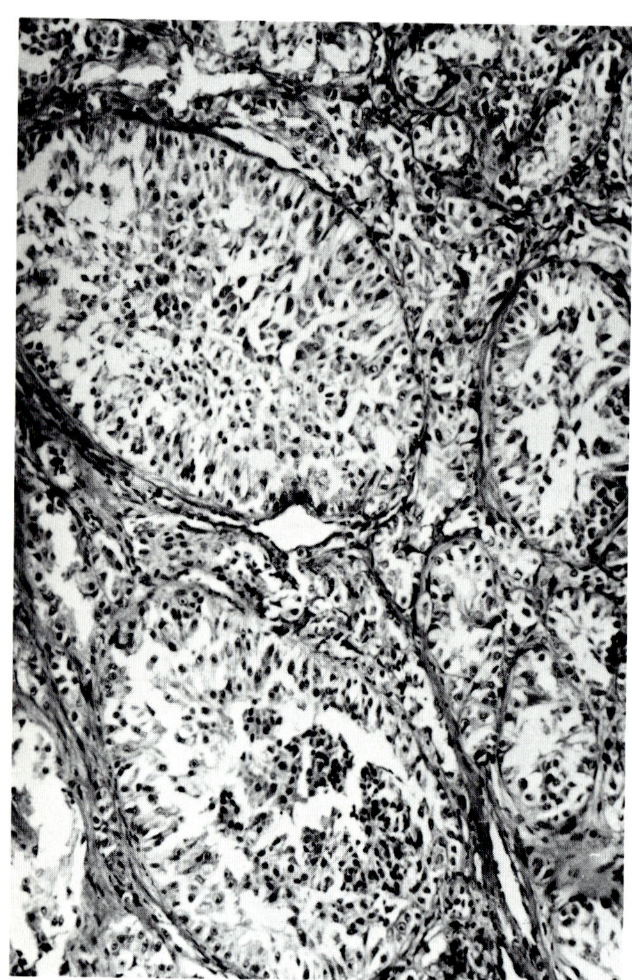

39.39 Sertoliform GCT of the ovary of an 8-year-old Spaniel bitch. ×127.

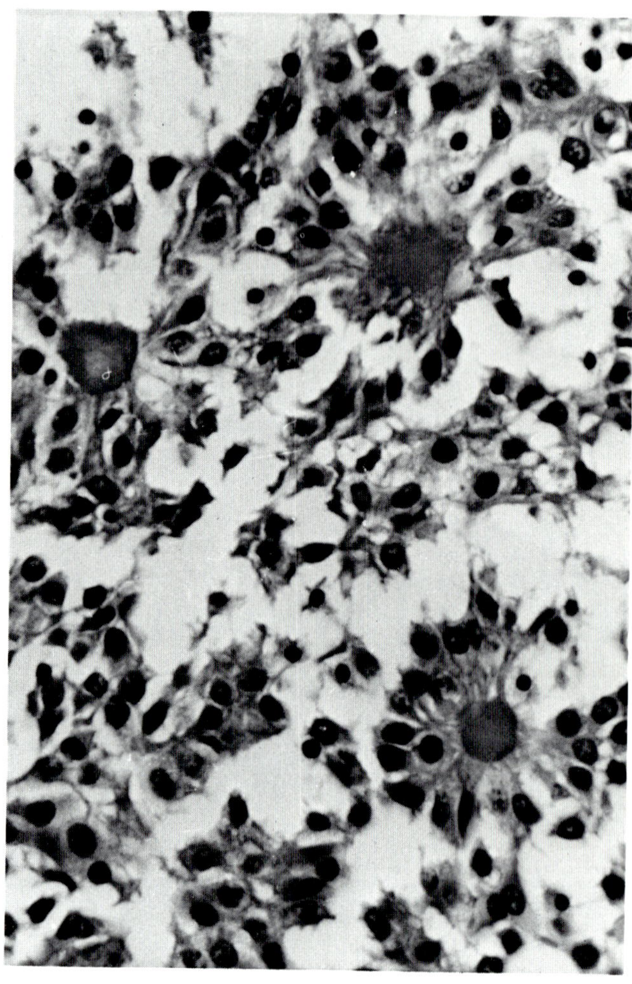

39.40 Call–Exner-like bodies in GCT of the ovary of a bitch (same tumor as Figure 39.37). ×813.

dometrial hyperplasia in one, and vaginal hemorrhage in one. Four of the Dehner et al.[47] dogs had a sanguinopurulent vaginal discharge.

The tumors had smooth, variably bulging surfaces and were of a gray, reddish, or bluish color with hemorrhagic areas. The typical tumor tissue was grayish white and rather soft, closely resembling the typical canine testicular seminoma.

On histologic examination, the tumors also resembled testicular seminomas. The tumor cells, which were large, rounded, angular, or polygonal, had large central chromatic nuclei, with a prominent nucleolus. The cytoplasm was eosinophilic or amphophilic or sometimes clear. Exceptionally large single nuclei and bi-, tri-, or multinucleated cells, as in canine testicular seminomas, were also seen. The resemblance was made still closer by the presence of clear spaces, often containing shrunken or ghost cells (Figure 39.42), and of spotty necrosis with karyorrhexis. Mitoses were numerous and sometimes abnormal.

The amount of stroma was usually small, and lymphocytic foci or granulomatous reactions were either not seen or were rare.[47]

Teratomas. Typical mature teratomas occur occasionally in dogs. Dehner et al.[47] described two instances, in dogs 2 and 8 years of age: One dog, which was emaciated, had an abdominal mass which on x ray films showed focal calcification; the other, with similar radiologic findings, also showed intermittent episodes of intestinal obstruction.

Storm[186] described a hair-bearing dermoid cyst 15 cm

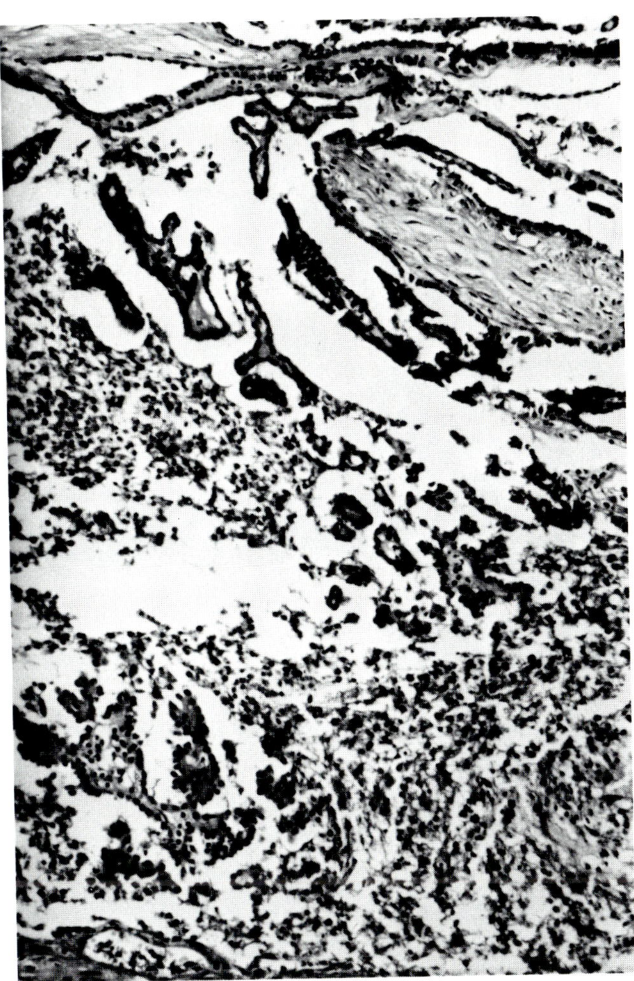

39.41 GCT of the ovary of an 8-year-old Spaniel bitch, showing diffuse granulosa cell areas and epithelial conformations. ×127.

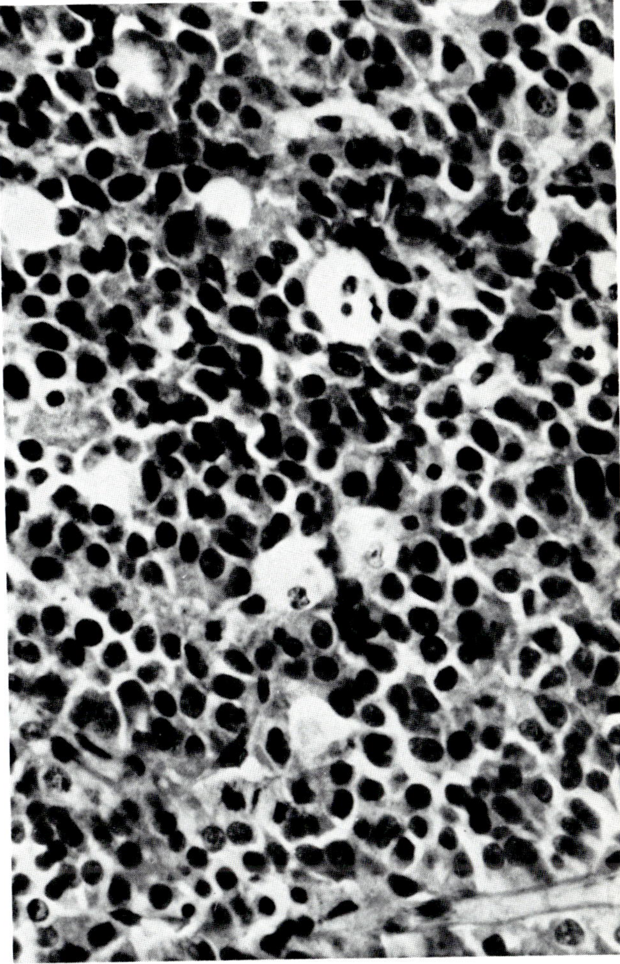

39.42 Seminoma of the ovary of a 10-year-old Scottish terrier bitch, showing multinucleate cells and clear spaces containing shrunken cells. ×813.

long in the left ovary of an 8-year-old Collie bitch and Riser et al.[170] described an almost equally large hair-bearing teratoma in the left ovary of a 5-year-old Pointer bitch. Benesch[19] found a teratoma filled with hair and weighing 2½ kg in the ovary of an 18-month-old Alsatian bitch. Röcken[171] has published a good account of a teratoma of the ovary in a 6-year-old Boxer bitch.

General discussion of canine ovarian tumors. There are three matters of interest raised by this study of canine ovarian tumors: first, their endocrine activity; second, their histogenesis; and third, their etiology. There is no doubt that some of these ovarian tumors are responsible for the hormonal effects that accompany their presence, for these signs regress when the tumors are surgically removed. However, a closer analysis of the particular hormones involved would be worthwhile. The indications are that the development of tumors of most kinds may lead to such conditions as pyometra, cystic endometrial hyperplasia, or vaginal hemorrhage. That such signs should accompany GCT is not surprising. Their relation to epithelial tumors and to dysgerminomas, however, is not easily understood, particularly in the latter instance.

As regards the histogenesis of canine ovarian tumors, it is not possible to give a completely satisfactory explanation. As a working hypothesis, however, I suggest the following: Papillomas, adenomas, papillary carcinomas, and adenocarcinomas are derived from the surface epithe-

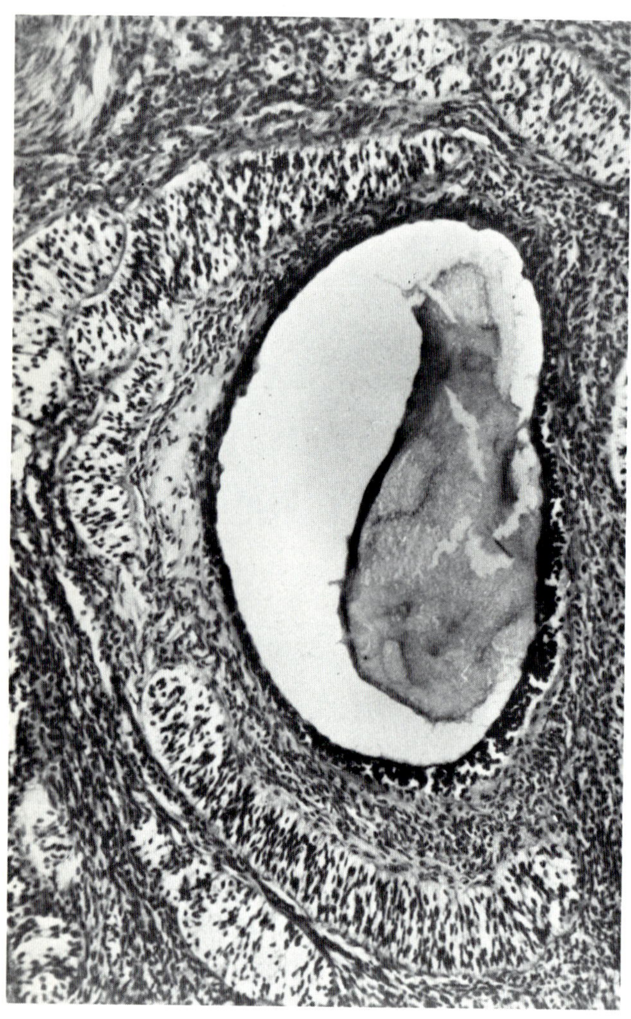

39.43 Sertoliform tubule around an atretic follicle in the ovary of a 12-year-old Miniature Poodle bitch. ×127.

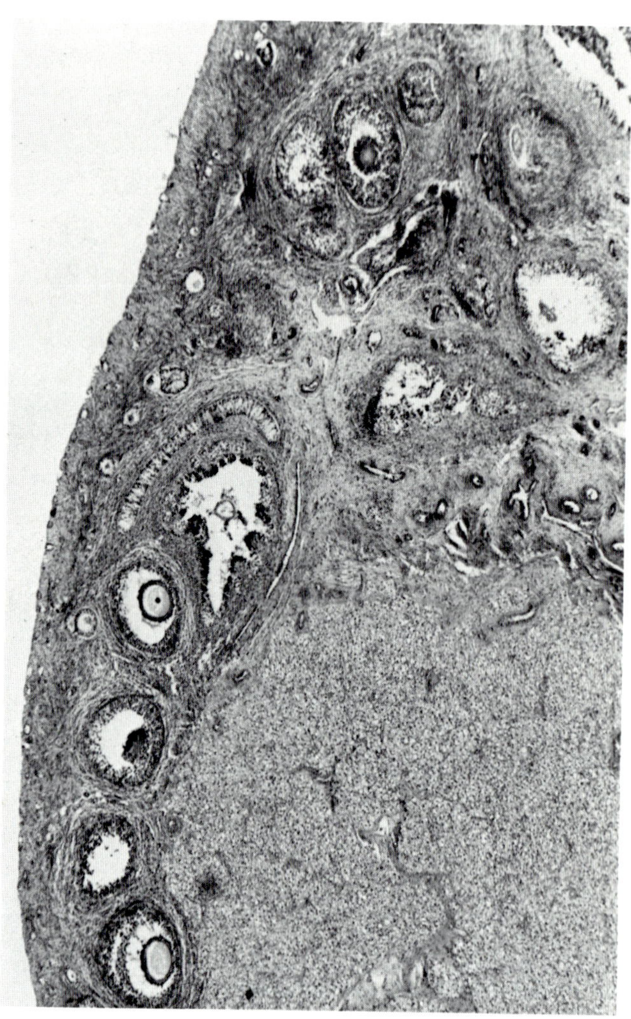

39.44 Part of the ovary of a 1-year-old Fox Terrier bitch, showing a Sertoliform tubule (left center) arching over a Graafian follicle, with a folded granulosa layer. ×32.

lium of the ovary, or from the epithelial cords that lie under the surface epithelium, or from both epithelia. In some of my tumors, the papillomatous conformation predominates, and it may be that these tumors are derived mainly if not wholly from the surface epithelium. However, some tumors appear to consist entirely of subsurface epithelial structures, and these may not contain a pure surface epithelial component.

There is some evidence for this view. Hormone-dependent epithelial proliferations were induced in bitches by the administration of diethylstilbestrol[104]; these lesions were reasonably interpretable as metastasizing carcinomas, some at least being hormone dependent. O'Shea and Jabara[158] produced histologic and histochemical evidence that these proliferative lesions were derived mainly from the surface epithelium but that some came from subsurface epithelial structures (SES), in which O'Shea had demonstrated characteristic sialic acid-containing mucinous secretion and intracytoplasmic droplets. O'Shea and Jabara[159] also found proliferative lesions of the serosa of the uterus in ovariectomized females treated with stilbestrol.

O'Shea and Jabara[158] were of the opinion that SES did not give rise to follicles, including oocytes, in adult dogs, but the coincident occurrence in canine ovarian tumors of tissues of undoubted granulosa cell origin and of epithelial tumor tissue with apparently smooth transitions between

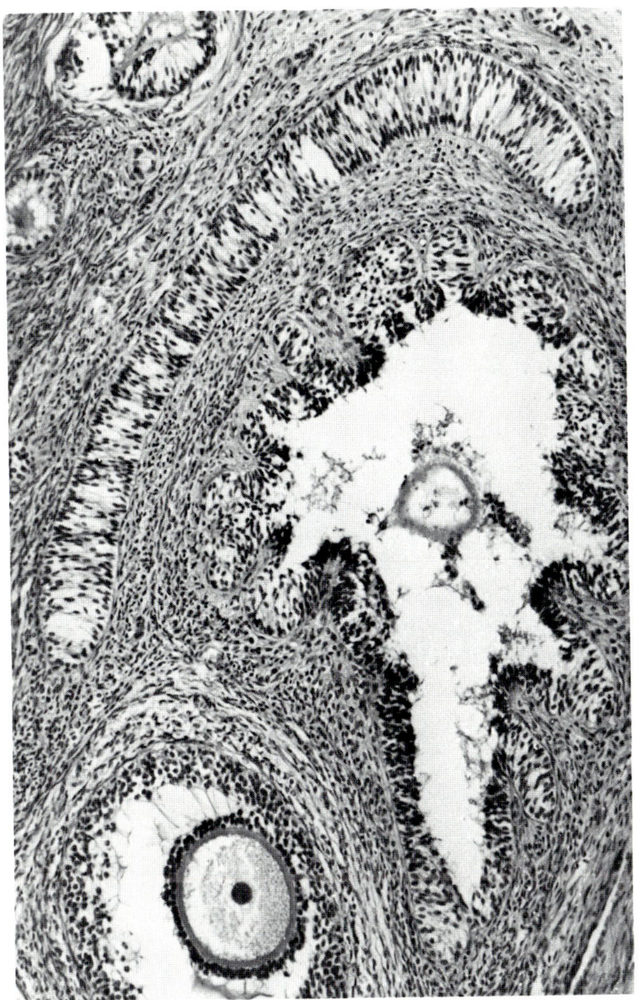

39.45 High power view of the Sertoliform tubule and follicle shown in Figure 39.44, showing apparent outward budding of granulosa layer. ×127.

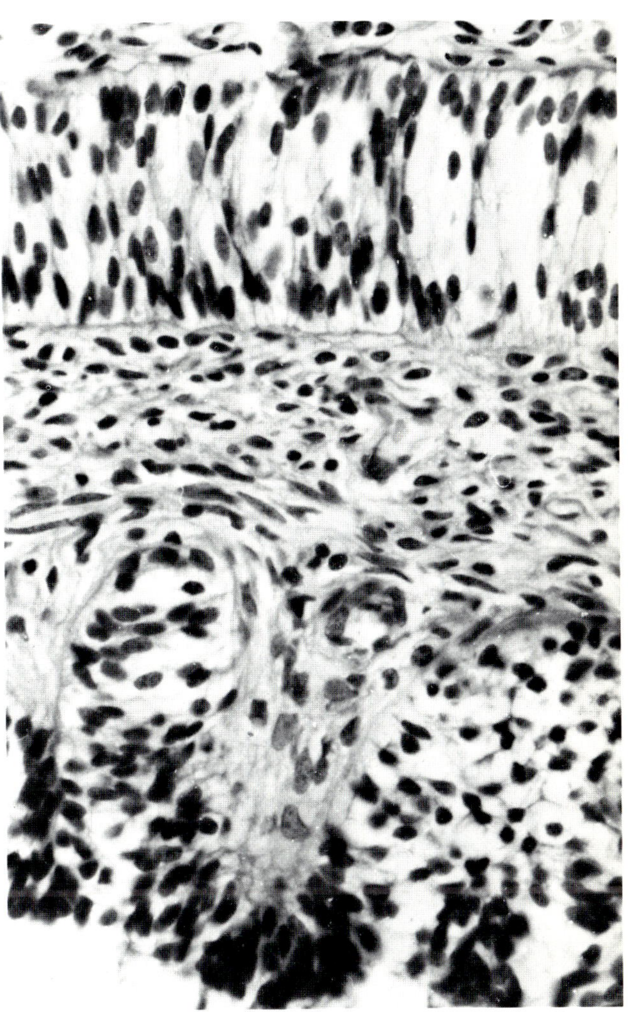

39.46 Closer view of the granulosa "buddings" and Sertoliform tubule seen in Figures 39.44 and 39.45. ×813.

the two, and also of tubular adenomas resembling the Sertoliform GCT in continuity with papillomas, suggests that the question needs further study.

As regards GCT, there is no difficulty in accepting that typical tumors are derived from the follicular granulosa layer. The problem is to account for the Sertoliform tumors, which are such a feature in the bitch but which are also found in man, cow, rat, and possibly other species. Anyone accustomed to examining the ovaries of the bitch will be struck by the common presence of small tubular structures, closely resembling immature testis tubules, lined by Sertoli-like cells (Figures 39.43 through 39.46). Sometimes these tubules are short and sometimes, in any one section, they are long. They occur at any level of the ovarian cortex and also in the hilus near the rete ovarii. Some are demonstrably continuous with the granulosa cell layer of follicles in which ova may still be present.

These tubules may partly be explained as being the "granulosa cell islands" described by Stott.[187] He states that germinal epithelial cells in the bitch are known to be mitotically active throughout life. Balls or cords of cells migrate into the cortex of the ovary from the germinal epithelium and, seemingly, invaginating germinal epithelial cells become granulosa cells. In the ovaries of 115 bitches, including 83 Beagles, ranging from 1 day to 19 years of age, he noted that at the appearance of the first signs of estrus (5 to 7 months of age) SES were seen in the outer cortex. Some SES had a lumen. Beneath the tunica albuginea, groups of SES containing primordial follicles were seen, as well as primary and growing follicles. Because many more follicles began to grow than reached maturity, follicular remnants were commonly seen in the ovary at this stage. From the fibroblast invasion of large atretic follicles, isolated granulosa cell islands (GCI) were formed. These GCI were more numerous in older bitches, especially those over 5 years old. It was noted that early or advanced proliferation of granulosa cells in GCI occurred, and this could result in GCT formation. Stott[187] illustrates tubular adenomas, one resembling a Sertoliform tumor, which could have arisen from SES.

Although this study by Stott[187] is very satisfying in providing an explanation of some Sertoliform GCT, the appearance in some canine ovaries of long Sertoli-like tubules is not easily directly attributable to follicular atresia; however, these tubules could of course have developed from GCI by a process of hyperplastic proliferation. Further study may show that at least some of these "testis cords" are, as defined by Mossman and Duke,[146] medullary cords persisting in adult ovaries and have the appearance of an immature seminiferous tubule or of the seminiferous tubule of a cryptorchid testis, but their possible relationship to "epithelial cords" derived from germinal epithelium (see Barton[16]) also needs study.

Dehner et al.[47] classify seminomas and teratomas as germ cell tumors and present a diagrammatic representation of their possible origin and relationship. They figure the dysgerminoma as a derivative of the primordial germ cells, which remains at the primordial level of histogenetic differentiation. A slight degree of differentiation produces an embryonal carcinoma (so far unidentified in dogs). From this stage trophoblastic differentiation would result in choriocarcinoma formation (so far unidentified in dogs), whereas somatic differentiation would result in the formation of a teratocarcinoma (so far unidentified in dogs), which, when completely differentiated, would form a mature teratoma (the typical form in the dog).

Summary

Inquiring readers will be able to pursue their studies further by reading in detail the various papers referred to in the references, but a few points are worth reemphasis.

In the case of uterine tumors, a striking fact is that carcinoma of the cervix is rarely reported in animals, and this is in accord with the concept that the cause of this cancer in women is likely to be specifically related to the human tumor. Again, if the apparent relative lack of bovine endometrial carcinomas in countries other than the United States can be confirmed, this may lead to a search for possible etiologic factors peculiar to that country. The apparent common occurrence of endometrial adenocarcinoma in some stocks of aged rabbits provides a useful model for study, for example, to search for a possible causal virus, or an unusual hormonal stimulus, or some specific genetic background. Similarly, the high incidence of carcinoma of the oviduct in domestic hens ought to facilitate the search for a possible causal agent or hormonal disturbance. Furthermore, the extreme rarity of endometrial choriocarcinoma in animals may be a significant "negative" observation.

In the case of ovarian tumors, there is an apparent important incidence of GCT in animals, and the not rare occurrence of this type of tumor in the bitch, for example, may permit more detailed hormonal and other functional analyses that may well have human relevance. Again, the occurrence of ovarian teratomas in Zebu cattle and in hares, for example, may facilitate histogenetic and other investigations of comparative medical importance.

If this chapter has alerted the medical oncologist to possible lines of inquiry in animals, it has served its purpose.

REFERENCES

1. Abraham, R. Equine ovarian teratoma. A case report. *Iowa State Univ. Vet. 30*:42, 1968.

2. Abrams, G. C. Diseases in an amphibian colony, *in* Mizell, M., ed.: *Biology of Amphibian Tumors.* New York, Springer-Verlag, 1965, p. 419.

3. Addis, M., and Baglioni, T. Sur un cas de cysto-adenoma papillaire de l'ovaire chez la chienne. *Proceedings of the 16th International Veterinary Congress 11*:271, 1959.

4. Amin, H. K., Ferenczy, A., and Richart, R. M. The ultrastructural features of a surface papilloma and serous cystadenofibroma respectively found incidentally in the ovaries of a two-year-old rhesus monkey. *J. Comp. Pathol. 84*:161, 1974.

5. Anderson, A. C. Carcinoma of the uterus in a Beagle. *J. Amer. Vet. Med. Assoc. 143*:500, 1963.

6. Anderson, L. J. and Sandison, A. T. Tumours of the female genitalia in cattle, sheep, and pigs found in a British abattoir survey. *J. Comp. Pathol. 79*:53, 1969.

7. Anderson, L. J., Sandison, A. T., and Jarrett, W. F. H. A British abattoir survey of tumours in cattle, sheep and pigs. *Vet. Rec. 84*:547, 1969.

8. Andervont, H. B., and Dunn, T. B. Occurrence of tumors in wild house mice. *J. Natl. Cancer Inst. 28*:1153, 1962.

9. Andrews, E. J., Stookey, J. L., Holland, D. R., and Slaughter, J. J. A histopathological study of canine and feline ovarian dysgerminomas. *Can. J. Comp. Med. 38*:85, 1974.

10. Appleby, E. C. Proceedings of the "Centennial Symposium on Science and Research" of the Philadelphia Zoological Society, November 1974 (in press).

11. Arbeiter, K. Der Scheidentumor bei der Hündin und seine operative Behandlung. *Wien. Tierärztl. Mschr. 48*:750, 1961.

12. Baba, N., and von Haam, E. Ultramicroscopic changes in the endometrial cells of spontaneous adenocarcinoma of rabbits. *J. Natl. Cancer Inst. 38*:657, 1967.

13. Baba, N., and von Haam, E. Spontaneous carcinoma in aged rabbits. *Am. J. Pathol. 68*:653, 1972.

14. Baker, E. Malignant granulosa cell tumor in a cat. *J. Am. Vet. Med. Assoc. 129*:322, 1956.

15. Balls, M. and Clothier, R. N. Spontaneous tumours in amphibia. *Oncology 29*:501, 1974.

16. Barton, E. P. The cyclic changes of epithelial cords in the dog ovary. *J. Morphol. 77*:317, 1945.

17. Baumann, R. Zur pathologischen Anatomie der Granulosazelltumoren des Eierstockes. *Wien. Tierärztl. Mschr. 22*:193, 1935.

18. Belter, I. F., Crawford, E. M., and Bates, H. R. Endometrial adenocarcinoma in a cat. *Pathol. Vet. 5*:429, 1968.

19. Benesch, F. 2½ Kg. schwere Dermoïdzyste des Ovariums bei einer Schäferhündin. *Wien. Tierärztl. Mschr. 22*:265, 1935.

20. Bielschowsky, M., and D'Ath, E. F. Spontaneous granulosa cell tumours in mice of strains NZC/B1, NZO/B1, NZY/B1 and NZO/B1. *Pathology 5*:303, 1973.

21. Brandly, P. J., and Migaki, G. Types of tumors found by Federal meat inspectors in an eight-year survey. *Ann. N.Y. Acad. Sci. 108*:872, 1963.

22. Brodey, R. S., and Roszel, J. F. Neoplasms of the canine uterus, vagina and vulva: A clinicopathologic survey of 90 cases. *J. Am. Vet. Med. Assoc. 151*:1294, 1967.

23. Buergelt, C. D. Dysgerminomas in two dogs. *J. Am. Vet. Med. Assoc. 153*:553, 1968.

24. Burghardt, R. Zur pathologischen Anatomie des Stuteneierstockes. *Arch. Wiss. Prakt. Tierheilk. 37*:455, 1911.

25. Burrows, H. Spontaneous uterine and mammary tumours in the rabbit. *J. Pathol. Bacteriol. 51*:385, 1940.

26. Campbell, J. G. Some unusual gonadal tumours of the fowl. *Br. J. Cancer 5*:69, 1951.

27. Campbell, J. G. *Tumours of the fowl.* London, Heinemann, 1909.

28. Carter, R. L. Pathology of ovarian neoplasms in rats and mice. *Eur. J. Cancer 3*:537, 1968.

29. Case, M. T., and Small, E. Ovarian carcinoma in a young dog. *Illinois Vet. 10*:6, 1967.

30. Chesterman, F. C., and Pomerance, A. Spontaneous neoplasms in ferrets and polecats. *J. Pathol. Bacteriol. 89*:529, 1965.

31. Chouroulinkov, I., Guillon, J. C., and Guérin, M. Endometrial sarcomas in mice: A survey of 130 cases. *J. Natl. Cancer Inst. 42*:593, 1969.

32. Christl, H. Ein angeborenes Ovarioblastom als Geburtshindernis. *Tierärztl. Umschau. 5*:276, 1950.

33. Christopher, J. Chorio-carcinoma in a bitch: A note. *Indian J. Anim. Sci. 42*:731, 1972.

34. Colombo, G. Neoformazione uterina nell cagna referible ad adenomiosi. *Zootec. e Vet. 19*:240, 1964.

35. Corcoran, C. J., and Murphy, E. C. Rare bovine placental tumour—a case report. *Vet. Rec. 77*:1234, 1965.

36. Cordes, D. O. Equine granulosa tumours. *Vet. Rec. 85*:186, 1969.

37. Cork, L. Ovarian cystadenocarcinoma in a bitch. *Southwest Vet. 23*:243, 1970.

38. Cotchin, E. Tumours of farm animals: A survey of tumours examined at the Royal Veterinary College during 1950–1960. *Vet. Rec. 72*:816, 1960.

39. Cotchin, E. Canine ovarian neoplasms. *Res. Vet. Sci. 2*:133, 1961.

40. Cotchin, E. Problems of comparative oncology with special reference to the veterinary aspects. *Bull. WHO 26*:633, 1962.

41. Cotchin, E. Spontaneous uterine tumours in animals. *Br. J. Cancer 18*:209, 1964.

42. Cotchin, E. Some aetiological aspects of tumours in domesticated animals. *Ann. R. Coll. Surg. Engl. 38*:92, 1966.

43. Cotchin, E. Comparative oncology. Neoplasms of domesticated animals of interest to medical and veterinary pathologists. *Pesquisa Agropecuaria, Brasileira, Série Veterinaria, 7*(Suppl.):1, 1972.

44. Crews, L. M., Kerber, W. T., and Feinman, H. An ovarian tumor of dual nature in a rhesus monkey. *Pathol. Vet. 4*:157, 1967.

45. Dämmrich, K., and Lettow, E. Adenokarzinom der Cervix uteri bei einer Hündin. *Berl. Münch. tierärztl. Wschr. 61*:51, 1968.

46. Davis, C. L., Leeper, R. S., and Shelton, J. E. Neoplasms encountered in federally inspected establishments in Denver, Colorado. *J. Am. Vet. Med. Assoc. 83*:229, 1933.

47. Dehner, L. P., Norris, H. J., Garner, F. M., and Taylor, H. B. Comparative pathology of ovarian neoplasms. III. Germ cell tumours of canine, bovine, feline, rodent and human species. *J. Comp. Pathol. 80*:299, 1970.

48. Deringer, M. K. Occurrence of tumors, particularly of mammary tumors, in agent-free strain C3HeB mice. *J. Natl. Cancer Inst. 22*:995, 1959.

49. Dewalque, J. Tumeur ovarienne et masculinisation chez une chèvre chamoisée. *Ann. Méd. Vét. 107*:322, 1963.

50. Di Domizio, G. Tumori ormonoattivi degli animali domestici. *Atti Soc. Ital. Sci. Vet. 1*:220, 1947.

51. Digiacomo, R. F., and McCann, T. O. Gynecologic pathology in the *Macaca mulatta*. Part I. *Am. J. Obstet. Gynecol. 108*:538, 1970.

52. Dorn, C. R., Taylor, D. O. N., and Chaulk, I. E. The prevalence of spontaneous neoplasms in a defined canine population. *Am. J. Public Health 56*:254, 1966.

53. Dorn, C. R., Taylor, D. O. N., and Frye, F. L. Survey of animal neoplasms in Alameda and Contra Costa Counties, California. I. Methodology and description of cases. *J. Natl. Cancer Inst. 40*:295, 1968.

54. Dorn, C. R., Taylor, D. O. N., Schneider, R., Hibbard, H. H., and Klauber, M. R. Survey of animal neoplasms in Alameda and Contra Costa Counties. II. Cancer morbidity in dogs and cats from Alameda County. *J. Natl. Cancer Inst. 40*:307, 1968.

55. Dow, C. Ovarian abnormalities in the bitch. *J. Comp. Pathol. 70*:59, 1960.

56. Drieux, H., and Le Coustumier. Hémangiome du chorion foetal chez la vache. *Rec. Méd. Vét. 142*:293, 1966.

57. Engle, E. T. Tubular adenoma and testis-like tubules of the ovaries of aged rats. *Cancer Res. 6*:578, 1946.

58. Fawcett, D. W. Bilateral ovarian teratomas in a mouse. *Cancer Res. 10*:705, 1950.

59. Federer, Otto. Über hormonal wirksame Ovarialblastome bei Hund und Katze. Inaugural-Dissertation, Berne, 1958, p. 24.

60. Fedrigo, M. Cistoadenocarcinoma papillare sieroso un-

differenziato dell'ovaio in una cagna. Aspetto clinico e terapeutico. *Veterinaria, 17*:22, 1968.

61. Fedrigo, M., and Rugiati, S. Alterazioni cromasomiche in une carcinoma ovarico di cagna. *Atti Soc. Ital. Sci. Vet. 21*:359, 1967.

62. Fekete, E., and Ferrigno, M. A. Studies on a transplantable teratoma of the mouse. *Cancer Res. 12*:438, 1952.

63. Feldman, G. B., Knapp, R. C., Order, S. E., and Hellman, S. The role of lymphatic obstruction in the formation of ascites in a murine ovarian carcinoma. *Cancer Res. 32*:1663, 1972.

64. Fessler, J. F., and Brobst, D. F. Granulosa cell tumor. *Cornell Vet. 62*:110, 1972.

65. Finckh, E. S. and Bolliger, A. Serous cystadenomata of the ovary in the koala. *J. Pathol. Bacteriol. 85*:526, 1963.

66. Finocchio, E. J., and Johnson, J. H. Granulosa cell tumor in a mare. *Vet. Med. 64*:322, 1969.

67. Flatt, R. E. Pyometra and uterine adenocarcinoma in a rabbit. *Lab. Anim. Care 19*:398, 1969.

68. Flux, J. E. C. Incidence of ovarian tumors in hares in New Zealand. *J. Wildlife Mgmt. 29*:622, 1965.

69. Fortner, J. G. Spontaneous tumors including gastrointestinal neoplasms and malignant melanomas in the Syrian hamster. *Cancer 10*:1153, 1957.

70. Fujimoto, Y., and Sakai, T. On a case of an ovarian cystadenoma associated with a teratoma(dermoid) in horse. *Jap. J. Vet. Res. 3*:8, 1955.

71. Fukushima, A., and Konishi, Y. A case report of feline ovarian tumor. *J. Jap. Vet. Med. Assoc. 23*:481, 1970.

72. Gardner, W. U., and Pan. S. C. Malignant tumors of the uterus and vagina in untreated mice of the PM stock. *Cancer Res. 8*:241, 1948.

73. Gardner, W. U., Strong, L. C., and Smith, G. M. An observation of primary tumors of the pituitary, ovaries and mammary glands in a mouse. *Am. J. Cancer 26*:541, 1936.

74. Gellatly, J. B. M. Normal and pathological anatomy and histology of the genital tract of rats and mice, *in* Cotchin, E., and Roe, F. C. J., eds.: *Pathology of Laboratory Rats and Mice.* Oxford and Edinburgh, Blackwell Scientific Publications, 1967, p. 498.

75. Gilmore, C. E. Tumors of the female reproductive tract. *Calif. Vet. 19*:12, 1965.

76. Goodchild, W. M. Personal communication, 1975.

77. Goodchild, W. M., and Cooper, D. M. Oviduct adenocarcinoma in laying hens. *Vet. Rec. 82*:389, 1968.

78. Goyon, M. Tératome ovarien avec métastases pulmonaires chez la hase. *Rec. Méd. Vét. 135*:651, 1959.

79. Grant, D. L. Uterine tumour in a mare—leio-myoma. *Vet. Rec. 76*:474, 1964.

80. Greene, H. S. N. Toxaemia of pregnancy in the rabbit. I. Clinical manifestations and pathology. *J. Exp. Med. 65*:809, 1937.

81. Greene, H. S. N. Toxaemia of pregnancy in the rabbit. II. Etiological considerations with special reference to hereditary factors. *J. Exp. Med. 67*:369, 1938.

82. Greene, H. S. N. Uterine adenomata in the rabbit. II. Homologous transplantation experiments. *J. Exp. Med. 69*:447, 1939.

83. Greene, H. S. N. Uterine adenomata in the rabbit. III. Susceptibility as a function of constitutional factors. *J. Exp. Med. 73*:273, 1941.

84. Greene, H. S. N. Diseases of the rabbit, in Ribelin, W. E. and McCoy, J. R., eds.: *The Pathology of Laboratory Animals.* Springfield, Charles C Thomas, 330, 1965.

85. Greene, H. S. N. and Newton, B. L. Evolution of cancer of the uterine fundus in the rabbit. *Cancer 1*:82, 1948.

86. Greene, H. S. N., Newton, B. L., and Fisk, A. A. Carcinoma of the vaginal wall in the rabbit. *Cancer Res. 7*:502, 1947.

87. Greene, H. S. N., and Saxton, J. A., Jr. Uterine adenomata in the rabbit. I. Clinical history, pathology and preliminary transplantation experiments. *J. Exp. Med. 67*:691, 1938.

88. Greene, H. S. N., and Strauss, J. S. Multiple primary tumors in the rabbit. *Cancer 2*:673, 1949.

89. Guarda, F. Contributo allo studio dei tumori ovarici. L'arrenoblastoma nella varietà di adenoma tubulare nel suino. *Ann. Fac. Med. Vet. Torino 8*:9, 1958.

90. Halloran, P. O'C. A bibliography of references to diseases in wild mammals and birds. *Am. J. Vet. Res. 16*(2):1, 1955.

91. Handler, A. H. Spontaneous lesions of the hamster, in Ribelin, W. E. and McCoy, J. R., eds.: *The Pathology of Laboratory Animals.* Springfield Ill. Charles C Thomas, 1965, p. 210.

92. Haranghy, L., Gyergyay, F., Antalffy, A., and Mérei, Gy. Meerschweinchentumoren. *Acta Morphol. 4*:301, 1954.

93. Hartigan, P. J., and Flynn, J. A. A scirrhous adenocarcinoma in the lungs of a slaughtered cow. *Irish Vet. J. 27*:161, 1973.

94. Hertig, A. T., and MacKey, J. J. Carcinoma *in situ* of the primate uterus: Comparative observations on the cervix of the crab-eating monkey, *Macaca fascicularis,* the endometrium of the chimpanzee, *Pan troglodytes,* and on similar lesions in the human patient. *Gynecol. Oncol. 1*:165, 1973.

95. Hilsdorf, L. Beitrag zur Kenntnis der Ovarialhyperplasien und—Geschwülste bei Rind, Schwein, Ziege und Hündin. *Münch. Tierärztl. Wschr. 77*:271, 1926.

96. Hisaw, F. L., and Hisaw, F. L., Jr. Spontaneous carcinoma of the cervix uteri in a monkey (*Macaca mulatta*). *Cancer 11*:810, 1958.

97. Hooker, C. W., and Strong, L. C. An ovarian tumor in a hermaphrodite mouse. *Cancer Res. 9*:550, 1949.

98. Horn, H. A., and Stewart, H. L. A review of some spontaneous tumors of noninbred mice. *J. Natl. Cancer Inst. 13*:591, 1952–1953.

99. Howard, F. A. Granulosa cell tumor of the equine ovary—a case report. *J. Am. Vet. Med. Assoc. 114*:134, 1949.

100. Iglesias, R., and Mardones, E. The influence of the gonads and of certain steroid hormones on the growth of the spontaneous and transplantable ovarian tumor in A × C rats. *Cancer Res. 16*:756, 1956.

101. Iglesias, R., Sternberg, W. H., and Segaloff, A. A functional ovarian tumor occurring spontaneously in a rat. *Cancer Res. 10*:226, 1950.

102. Ingalls, T. H., Adams, W. M., Lurie, M. B., and Ipsen, J. Natural history of adenocarcinoma of the uterus in the Phipps rabbit colony. *J. Natl. Cancer Inst. 33*:799, 1964.

103. Ishmael, J. Dysgerminoma of the ovary in a bitch. *J. Small Anim. Pract. 11*:697, 1970.

104. Jabara, A. G. Induction of canine ovarian tumours by diethylstilboestrol and progesterone. *Aust. J. Exp. Biol. Med. Sci. 40*:139, 1962.

105. Jackson, E. B., and Brues, A. M. Studies on a transplantable embryoma of the mouse. *Cancer Res. 1*:494, 1941.

106. Jacobs, B. B., and Huseby, R. A. Neoplasms occurring in aged Fischer rats, with special reference to testicular, uterine and thyroid tumors. *J. Natl. Cancer Inst.* *39*:303, 1967.

107. Jain, S. K., Singh, D. K., and Rae, U. R. K. Granulosa cell tumour in a guinea pig. *Indian Vet. J.* *47*:563, 1970.

108. Jennings, A. R. Tumours of free-living wild mammals and birds in Great Britain. *Symp. Zool. Soc. Lond.* No. 24, 273, 1968.

109. Joshi, K. V., Sardeshpande, P. D., Jalnapurkar, B. V., and Ajinkyo, S. M. A case of uterine adenocarcinoma in a dog. *Indian Vet. J.* *44*:114, 1967.

110. Kanagawa, H., Kawata, K., Nakao, N., and Sung, W. K. A case of granulosa cell tumor of the ovary in a newborn calf. *Jap. J. Vet. Res.* *12*:7, 1964.

111. Karetta, F. Über ein skirrhöses Karzinom des Uterus beim Rind. *Wien. Tierärztl. Mschr.* *15*:625, 1928.

112. Karlson, A. G., and Kelly, M. D. Choriohemangioma of the bovine allantois-chorion. *J. Am. Vet. Med. Assoc.* *99*:133, 1941.

113. Keindorf, H. J. Ein Uterusmischgeschwulst beim Rind-Ätiologische und differentialdiagnostische Betrachtungen. *Mh. Vet. Med.* *26*:522, 1971.

114. King, R. C. Hereditary ovarian tumors of *Drosophila melanogaster,* in C. J. Dawe and J. C. Harshberger, eds.: *Neoplasms and Related Disorders of Invertebrates and Lower Vertebrate Animals,* Monograph 31. Washington, D.C., Natl. Cancer Inst., 1969, p. 323.

115. Kirkbride, C. A., Bicknell, E. J., and Robl, M. G. Hemangiomas of a bovine fetus with chorioangioma of the placenta. *Vet. Pathol.* *10*:238, 1973.

116. Kraemer, D. C., and Vera Cruz, N. C. The female reproductive system, in R. N. T.-W.-Fiennes, ed.: *Pathology of Simian Primates.* Part 1: *General Pathology.* Karger, Basel, 1972, p. 841.

117. Kronberger, H. Spontane Geschwülste bei Haussäugetieren. *Mh. Vet. Med.* *15*:730, 1961.

118. Kullander, S. Studies on spayed rats with ovarian tissue autotransplanted into the spleen. *Acta Endocrinol.* *24*:307, 1957.

119. Lagerlöf, N., and Boyd, H. Ovarian hypoplasia and other abnormal conditions in the sexual organs of cattle of the Swedish Highland breed: Results of post-mortem examination of over 6,000 cows. *Cornell Vet.* *43*:64, 1953.

120. Leopold, A. Tumore a cellule della granulosa dell'ovaio destro in una cavalla. *Nuova Vet.* *43*:168, 1967.

121. Lindsey, J. R., Wharton, L. R., Woodruff, J. D., and Baker, H. J. Intrauterine choriocarcinoma in a rhesus monkey. *Path. Vet.* *6*:378, 1969.

122. Lingard, D. R., and Dickinson, E. O. Uterine adenocarcinoma with metastasis in the cow. *J. Am. Vet. Med. Assoc.* *148*:913, 1966.

123. Lingeman, C. H. Etiology of cancer of the human ovary: A review. *J. Natl. Cancer Inst.* *53*:1603, 1974.

124. Lipschutz, A., Iglesias, R., Rojas, G., and Cerisola, H. Spontaneous tumorigenesis in aged guinea-pigs. *Br. J. Cancer* *13*:486, 1959.

125. Loeb, L. Ueber chorionepitheliomartige Gebilde im Ovarium des Meerschweinchens und über ihre wahrscheinliche Entstehung aus parthogenetisch sich entwickelnden Eiern. *Z. Krebsforsch.* *11*:259, 1912.

126. Lombard, C. Nouvelle observation de cancer utérin chez la lapine. *Bull. Acad. Vét. Fr.* *32*:447, 1959.

127. Lombard, C. Contribution à l'étude des tumeurs de l'appareil génital, chez les mammifères domestiques. *Rev. Méd. Vét.* *112*:509 and 598, 1961.

128. Lombard, C. Deux cas de tumeurs de gibier. *Bull. Acad. Vét. Fr.* *35*:39, 1962.

129. Lombard, C., and Havet, J. Premier cas de seminoma ovarien chez la truie. *Bull. Acad. Vét. Fr.* *35*:135, 1962.

130. Maeda, T., Hayashi, T., Sasaki, H., and Tsumura, I. Tumors of the genital organs in domestic animals. I. Uterine and vaginal tumors in cows and a sow. *J. Jap. Vet. Med. Assoc.* *24*:226, 1971.

131. Maeda, T., Tsumura, I., Sasaki, H., Osugi, T., Omura, Y., and Kido, H. Tumors of genital organs in domestic animals. II. Seven cases of ovarian tumors in cows and sows. *J. Jap. Vet. Med. Assoc.* *26*:134, 1973.

132. Malinin, G. I., and Malinin, I. M. Age-related spontaneous uterine lesions in mice. *J. Gerontol.* *27*:193, 1972.

133. Marin-Padilla, M. and Benirschke, K. Thalidomide induced alterations in the blastocyst and placenta of the armadillo, *Dasypus novemcinctus mexicanus,* including a choriocarcinoma. *Am. J. Pathol.* *43*:999, 1963.

134. Martin, C. B. Jr., Misenhimer, H. R., and Ramsey, E. M. Ovarian tumors in rhesus monkeys (*Macaca mulatta*): Report of three cases. *Lab. Anim. Care* *20*:686, 1970.

135. Mastronardi, M., and Potena, A. Contributo alla conoscenze dei tumori ovarici nella cavalla. *Acta Med. Vet.* *12*:171, 1966.

136. Mawdesley-Thomas, L. E. An ovarian tumour in a southern elephant seal (*Mirounga leonina*). *Vet. Pathol.* *8*:9, 1971.

137. Mawdesley-Thomas, L. E., and Bonner, W. N. Uterine tumours in a grey seal (*Halichoerus grypus*). *J. Pathol.* *103*:205, 1971.

138. McCann, T. O., and Myers, R. E. Endometriosis in rhesus monkeys. *Am. J. Obstet. Gynecol.* *106*:516, 1970.

139. Meier, H. Carcinoma of the uterus in the cat: Two cases. *Cornell Vet.* *46*:188, 1956.

140. Meissner, W. A., Sommers, S. C., and Sherman, G. Endometrial hyperplasia, endometrial carcinoma, and endometriosis produced experimentally by estrogen. *Cancer* *10*:500, 1957.

141. Migaki, G., Carey, A. M., Turnquest, R. U., and Garner, F. M. Pathology of bovine uterine adenocarcinoma. *J. Am. Vet. Med. Assoc.* *157*:1577, 1970.

142. Misdorp, W. Tumours in large domestic animals in the Netherlands. *J. Comp. Pathol.* *77*:211, 1967.

143. Monlux, A. W., Anderson, W. A., Davis, C. L., and Monlux, W. S. Adenocarcinoma of the uterus of the cow—differentiation of its pulmonary metastases from primary lung tumors. *Am. J. Vet. Res.* *17*:45, 1956.

144. Moreland, A. F., and Woodard, J. C. A spontaneous uterine tumor in a New World primate *Saguinus* (*Oedipomidas*) *oedipus. Pathol. Vet.* *5*:193, 1968.

145. Mosinger, M. Sur la carcinorésistance du cobaye. Première partie. Les tumeurs spontanées du cobaye. *Bull. Assoc. Franc. Cancer* *48*:235, 1961.

146. Mossman, H. W., and Duke, K. L. *Comparative Morphology of the Mammalian Ovary.* Madison, University of Wisconsin Press, 1973.

147. Murphy, E. D. Hyperplastic and early neoplastic changes

in the ovaries of mice after genetic deletion of germ cells. *J. Natl. Cancer Inst.* *48*:1283, 1972.

148. Murphy, E. D., and Beamer, W. G. Plasma gonadotropin levels during early stages of ovarian tumorigenesis in mice of the W^x/W^v genotype. *Cancer Res.* *33*:721, 1973.

149. Nelson, L. W., Todd, G. G., and Migaki, G. Ovarian neoplasms in swine. *J. Amer. Vet. Med. Assoc.* *151*:1331, 1967.

150. Noordsy, J. L., Leipold, H. W., Cook, J. E., and Downing, C. W. Leiomyosarcoma of the uterus in a Holstein cow. *Vet. Med.* *68*:176, 1973.

151. Norris, H. J., Garner, F. M., and Taylor, H. B. Pathology of feline ovarian neoplasms. *J. Pathol.* *97*:138, 1969.

152. Norris, H. J., Garner, F. M. and Taylor, H. B. Comparative pathology of ovarian neoplasms. IV. Gonadal stromal tumours of canine species. *J. Comp. Pathol.* *80*:399, 1970.

153. Norris, H. J., Taylor, H. B., and Garner, F. M. Equine ovarian granulosa tumours. *Vet. Rec.* *82*:419, 1968.

154. Norris, H. J., Taylor, H. B., and Garner, F. M. Comparative pathology of ovarian neoplasms. II. Gonadal stromal tumors of bovine species. *Pathol. Vet.* *6*:45, 1969.

155. Nowotny, F. Granulosazelltumor bei einem Eichhörnchen (*Sciurus vulgaris* L.) *Wien. Tierärztl. Mschr.* *49*:158, 1962.

156. O'Gara, R. W., and Adamson, R. H. Spontaneous and induced neoplasms in nonhuman primates, *in* R. N. T.-W.-Fiennes, ed.: *Pathology of Simian Primates.* Part 1. General Pathology. Basel, Karger, 1972, p. 190.

157. O'Rourke, M. D., and Geib, L. W. Endometrial adenocarcinoma in a cat. *Cornell Vet.* *60*:598, 1970.

158. O'Shea, J. D., and Jabara, A. G. The histogenesis of canine ovarian tumours induced by stilboestrol administration. *Pathol. Vet.* *4*:137, 1967.

159. O'Shea, J. D., and Jabara, A. G. Proliferative lesions of serous membranes in ovariectomised female and entire male dogs after stilboestrol administration. *Vet. Pathol.* *8*:81, 1971.

160. Ottosen, H. E. Scirrhøse adenokarcinomer i Uterus hos Køer. *Skand. Vet. Tidskr.* *33*:473, 1943.

161. Parodi, A. L. *Tumeurs spontanées de l'ovaire chez l'animal. Revue Générale.* Extrait des XXVIIes Assises Françaises de Gynécologie sur Les Tumeurs de l'Ovaire. Masson et Cie, Paris, 1975, p. 7.

162. Polding, J. B., and Lall, H. K. Some genital abnormalities of the Indian cow and buffalo with reference to anatomical differences in their genital organs. *Indian J. Vet. Sci.* *15*:178, 1945.

163. Polson, C. J. Tumours of the rabbit. *J. Pathol. Bacteriol.* *30*:603, 1927.

164. Preiser, H. Endometrial adenocarcinoma in a cat. *Pathol. Vet.* *1*:485, 1964.

165. Priester, S. W., and Mantel, N. Occurrence of tumors in domestic animals. Data from 12 United States and Canadian Colleges of Veterinary Medicine. *J. Natl. Cancer Inst.* *47*:1333, 1971.

166. Rewell, R. E. Uterine fibromas and bilateral ovarian granulosa-cell tumours in a senile squirrel monkey, *Saimiri sciurea. J. Pathol. Bacteriol.* *68*:291, 1954.

167. Rewell, R. E., and Willis, R. A. Some tumours found in whales. *J. Pathol. Bacteriol.* *61*:454, 1949.

168. Riedel, W. Ein metastasierendes Uteruskarzinom einer Ziege. *Berl. Münch. Tierärztl. Wschr.* *77*:395, 1964.

169. Rigdon, R. H. Tumors in the duck (family Anatidae): A review. *J. Natl. Cancer Inst.* *49*:467, 1972.

170. Riser, W. H., Marcus, J. F., Guibor, E. C., and Oldt, C. C. Dermoid cyst of the canine ovary. *J. Am. Vet. Med. Assoc.* *134*:27, 1959.

171. Röcken, H. Bildbericht: Teratombildung und gleichzeitige Trächtigkeit beim Hund. *Berl. Münch. Tierärztl. Wschr.* *86*:74, 1973.

172. Rogers, J. B., and Blumenthal, H. T. Studies of guinea-pig tumors. I. Report of fourteen spontaneous guinea-pig tumors with a review of the literature. *Cancer Res.* *20*:191, 1960.

173. Rowe, S. E., Simmons, J. L., Ringler, D. H., and Lay, D. M. Spontaneous neoplasms in aging Gerbillinae. A summary of forty-four neoplasms. *Vet. Pathol.* *11*:38, 1974.

174. Russell, E. S., and Fekete, E. Analysis of W-series pleiotropism in the mouse. Effect of W^vW^v substitution on definitive germ cells and on ovarian tumorigenesis. *J. Natl. Cancer Inst.* *21*:365, 1958.

175. Russfield, A. B. Pathology of the endocrine glands, ovary and testis of rats and mice, *in* Cotchin, E. and Roe, F. C. J., eds.: *Pathology of Laboratory Rats and Mice.* Oxford and Edinburgh, Blackwell Scientific Publications, 1967, p. 391.

176. Sbernardori, U., and Nava, A. Disgerminoma dell'ovaio nella gatta. *Clin. Vet. Milano* *91*:333, 1968.

177. Schardein, J. L., Fitzgerald, J. E., and Kaump, D. H. Spontaneous tumors in Holtzman-source rats of various ages. *Path. Vet.* *5*:238, 1968.

178. Scheuler, R. L., and Ediger, R. Murine ovarian teratoma. *Amer. J. Vet. Res.* *36*:341, 1975.

179. Schlegel, M. Bedeutung, Vorkommen, und Charakteristik der Ovarialtumoren bei den Haustieren. *Berl. Tierärztl. Wschr.* *31*:589, 1915.

180. Schulze, F. Spontantumoren der Schädelhöhle und Genitalorgane bei Sprague–Dawley und Bethesda-Black Ratten. *Z. Krebsforsch.* *64*:78, 1968.

181. Sedlmeier, H. Drei bemerkenswerte Fälle von Uterustumoren. *Münch. Tierärztl. Wschr.* *81*:89, 1930.

182. Seibold, H. R., and Wolf, R. H. Neoplasms and proliferative lesions in 1065 nonhuman primate necropsies. *Lab. Anim. Sci.* *23*:533, 1973.

183. Short, R. V., Shorter, D. R., and Linzell, J. L. Granulosa cell tumour of the ovary in a virgin heifer. *J. Endocrinol.* *27*:327, 1963.

184. Snell, K. Spontaneous lesions of the rat, *in* Ribelin, W. E., and McCoy, J. R., eds.: *The Pathology of Laboratory Animals.* Springfield, Ill., Charles C Thomas, 1965, p. 241–300.

185. Sternberg, S. S. Carcinoma *in situ* of the cervix in a monkey (*Macaca mulatta*). *Amer. J. Obstet. Gynecol.* *82*:96, 1961.

186. Storm, R. E. Dermoid cyst of the ovary. *N. Am. Vet.* *28*:30, 1947.

187. Stott, G. G. Granulosa-cell islands in the canine ovary: Histogenesis, histopathologic features, and fate. *Am. J. Vet. Res.* *35*:1351, 1974.

188. Streett, J. J. A note on a teratoma occurring in the Leopard frog. *Tex. J. Sci.* *16*:493, 1964.

189. Strong, L. C., Gardner, W. U., and Hill, R. T. Production of estrogenic hormone by a transplantable ovarian carcinoma. *Endocrinology* *21*:269, 1937.

190. Strozier, L. M., McClure, H. M., Keeling, M. E., and

Cummins, L. B. Endometrial adenocarcinoma, endometriosis, and pyometra in a rhesus monkey. *J. Am. Vet. Med. Assoc. 161*:704, 1972.

191. Studer, E. Mucinous adenocarcinoma of the bovine ovary. *J. Am. Vet. Med. Assoc. 151*:438, 1967.

192. Summers, P. M. An abattoir study of the genital pathology of cows in Northern Australia. *Aust. Vet. J. 50*:403, 1974.

193. Symeonidis, A., and Mori-Chavez, P. A. A transplantable ovarian papillary adenocarcinoma of the rat with ascites implants in the ovary. *J. Natl. Cancer Inst. 13*:409, 1952–1953.

194. Taylor, D. O. N., and Dorn, C. R. Dysgerminoma in a 20-year-old female German Shepherd dog. *Am. J. Vet. Res. 28*:587, 1967.

195. Terlecki, A., and Watson, W. A. Adenocarcinoma of the uterus of a ewe. *Vet. Rec. 80*:516, 1967.

196. Teutscher, R. Ein Plattenepithelkrebs der Schamlippe der Stute. *Dtsch. Tierärztl. Wschr. 66*:567, 1959.

197. Thiery, M. Ovarian teratoma in the mouse. *Br. J. Cancer 17*:231, 1963.

198. Thompson, S. W., and Hunt, R. D. Spontaneous tumors in the Sprague-Dawley rat. *Ann. N.Y. Acad. Sci. 108*:832, 1963.

199. Thompson, S. W., Huseby, R. A., Fox, M. A., Davis, C. L., and Hunt, R. D. Spontaneous tumors in the Sprague-Dawley rat. *J. Natl. Cancer Inst. 27*:1037, 1961.

200. Trotter, A. M. Carcinoma of the uterus of a cow. *J. Comp. Pathol. 19*:41, 1906.

201. Trotter, A. M. Malignant diseases in bovines. *J. Comp. Pathol. 24*:1, 1911.

202. Vandeplasche, M. and Thoonen, J. Reuze tumoren in de baarmoeder bij een koe. *Vlaam. Diergeneesk. Tijdschr. 19*:157, 1950.

203. Vink, H. H. Ovarian teratomas in guineapigs. A report of ten cases. *J. Pathol. 102*:180, 1970.

204. Ward, B. C., and Moore, W., Jr. Spontaneous lesions in a colony of Chinese hamsters, *Cricetulus griseus. Lab. Anim. Care 19*:516, 1969.

205. Warren, S., and Gates, O. Spontaneous and induced tumors of the guinea pig. *Cancer Res. 1*:65, 1941.

206. Weir, B. J. Some observations on reproduction in the female agouti. *J. Reprod. Fertil. 24*:203, 1971.

207. Weisbroth, S. H. Neoplastic diseases, in Weisbroth, S. H., Flatt, R. E., and Kraus, A. L. eds.: *The Biology of the Laboratory Rabbit.* New York, Academic Press, 1974, Ch. 14, 331.

208. West, J. L. Arrhenoblastoma in a chukar partridge. *Avian Dis. 18*:258, 1974.

209. Weston, J. K. Spontaneous lesions in monkeys, in Ribelin, W. E., and McCoy, J. B., eds.: *The Pathology of Laboratory Animals.* Springfield, Ill., Charles C Thomas, 1965, p. 351.

210. Whiteley, H. J., and Horton, D. L. A spontaneous transplantable ovarian tumour of the CBA mouse. *Br. J. Cancer 17*:252, 1964.

211. Wilcox, D. E., and Mossman, H. W. The common occurrence of "testis" cords in the ovaries of a shrew (*Sorex vagrans*, Baird). *Anat. Rec. 92*:183, 1945.

212. Willis, R. A. Ovarian teratomas in guineapigs. *J. Pathol. Bacteriol. 84*:237, 1962.

213. Winterfeldt, K. V. Ein Leiomyom des Ligamentum latum uteri eines Schweines. *Dtsch. Tierärztl. Wschr. 71*:70, 1964.

214. World Health Organization. International histological classification of tumours of domestic animals. *Bull. WHO 50*:1, 1974.

215. Wurster, A. C. Granulosa cell tumor in the ovary of a mare. *Southwest Vet. 17*:149, 1964.

216. Wyssmann, E. Uteruskrebs als Ursache der Nichtöffnung des Cervix uteri int. bein einer Kälbin. *Schweiz. Archiv. Tierheilk. 54*:8, 1912.

217. Yamauchi, S. A histological study of ovaries of aged cows. *Jap. J. Vet. Sci. 25*:315, 1963.

218. Yang, Y. H. Endometrial metaplasia in an albino rat. *Pathol. Vet. 1*:491, 1964.

219. Zaldivar, R. Incidence of spontaneous neoplasms in beagles. *J. Am. Vet. Med. Assoc. 151*:1319, 1967.

Index

Aardwolf, uterine tumors in, 32
Abattoir surveys, of genital tract tumors, 27, 32, 33, 37, 44
A × C rats
  ovarian tumors in, 7, 39
  uterine tumors in, 15
2-Acetylaminofluorene, *see* 2-Fluorenylacetamide
ACI rats, ovarian tumors in, 39
Adenoacanthomas
  in domestic animals, 45
  of uterus, 15, 19
Adenocarcinoma(s)
  of cervix, 19
  in domestic animals, 28, 29, 32–34, 45, 49, 53, 57–58, 60
  in laboratory animals, 5, 31, 34–38, 40
  of uterus, 13–15
  of vagina, afternatal stilbestrol therapy, 17
Adenofibromyomas, of uterus, 14
Adenomas
  in domestic animals, 28, 50–52, 57–58, 60
  in laboratory animals, 4, 6, 9, 35, 38–40
  in wild animals, 42
Adenomatous hyperplasia, of endocervical glands, in monkeys, 29
Adenomatous polyps, in laboratory animals, 31
Adenomyomas, in laboratory animals, 31
β-Adrenergic receptor stimulants, ovarian tumor induction by, 5
Agouti
  ovarian tumors in, 41
  uterine tumors in, 31
Alsatian
  ovarian tumors in, 52-55, 57
  uterine tumors in, 28
β-Aminoazotoluene, ovarian tumor induction by, 5
Anas platyrhynchos, see Mallard duck
Androblastomas, in laboratory animals, 39
Androgens
  ovarian tumor induction by, 8
  uterine tumor induction by, 14
Angiosarcomas, in laboratory animals, 31
Angora rabbits, uterine tumors in, 36
Animal models
  criteria for use of, 1–2
  for ovarian and uterine tumors, 1–25
  for tumors of cervix, vagina, and vulva, 16–20
Antelope, uterine tumors in, 31
Armadillo
  choriocarcinoma in, 30
  uterine tumors in, 31
Arrhenoblastomas
  in domestic animals, 37, 49
  in laboratory animals, 39
  in wild animals, 42
Atresia, of oocytes in mouse, 2
Axis deer, uterine tumors in, 31

Baboons, herpes infections of, 19
Balaenoptera sp., *see* Whale
BALB/c mice
  cervical cancer in, 17

BALB/c mice [*cont.*]
ovarian tumors in, 3, 8, 11
uterine tumors in, 13
vaginal tumors in, 19
BC mice, vaginal tumors in, 17
Beagle
ovarian tumors in, 49–50
subsurface epithelial structures in ovary of, 58
uterine tumor in, 28
Benzo[*a*]pyrene
ovarian tumor induction by, 5
vaginal tumor induction by, 17
Birds, ovarian tumors in, 40–43
Blesbok, uterine tumors in, 31
Blue whale, ovarian tumors in, 41
Bontebok, uterine tumors in, 31
Bos taurus, see Cow
Boxer, ovarian tumor in, 57
Brahman cattle, ovarian tumors in, 46–49
Brenner ovarian tumor, in animals, 14, 49
Broiler chickens, ovarian tumors in, 49
BUF rats, ovarian tumors in, 39
Buffalo, uterine tumors in, 38
Buffalo strain rats, uterine tumors in, 15
Bulldog, ovarian tumor in, 54
N-Butyl-*N*-nitrosourea, placental tumor induction by, 16

Call-Exner bodies, in ovarian tumors, 48, 55, 56
Canis familiaris, see Dog
Capra hircus, see Goat
Carbowax 1000, vaginal and cervical tumor induction by, 19
Carcinoleiomyosarcoma, in domestic animal, 29
Carcinoma(s). (*See also* Squamous cell carcinomas)
of cervix, 16, 17
in domestic animals, 32–37, 44–46, 50
in situ, in laboratory primate, 30
in laboratory animals, 30, 31, 39
of ovary, 9, 39, 42, 44–46, 50
of vagina, 17
in wild and zoo mammals, 31, 42
Carcinosarcomas, of salivary glands, from chemical carcinogens, 15
Cats
ovarian tumors in, 4, 9, 47–49
tumors in, classification, 27
uterine tumors in, 28, 29
C57B1 mice, ovarian tumors in, 10, 11
CBA mice
oocyte atresia in, 2
ovarian tumors in, 3, 6, 11, 38
uterine tumors in, 13–15
CE mice, ovarian tumors in, 6, 38
Cebus monkeys
herpes infections of, 19
ovarian tumors in, 38
Cervix
in animals, 2, 12
animal models for tumors of, 16–20
perinatal changes in, 12
sex hormone effects on, 13
tumors of, 20, 27, 60
in domesticated animals, 34
in wild animals, 32
C3H mice
cervical tumors in, 18
ovarian tumors in, 6, 38
induced, 4, 10, 11
uterine tumors in, 13
Chamois goat, ovarian tumor in, 41
Charadiformes, ovarian tumors in, 42
Charles River CD rats, ovarian tumors in, 5
Chemical carcinogens
ovarian tumor induction by, 4–5, 12
placental tumor induction by, 16
uterine tumor induction by, 14–15, 20
Chickens, *see* Fowl
Chondrosarcoma, in laboratory animals, 39
Chorioadenoma destruens, induced placental tumor resembling, 16
Choriocarcinomas, 60
induction of, 16
spontaneous, 27, 30
Choriohemangioma, in cow, 34
Chorioma, in wild animals, 31
Chorionic epithelioma, in wild animals, 31
Chukar partridge, ovarian tumor in, 42–43
Cobalt-60, uterine tumor induction by, 15
Cocker spaniel, ovarian tumor in, 56, 57
Collie, ovarian tumor in, 57
Computer, use in animal tumor survey, 27
Contraceptives, intravaginal, animal tumor induction by, 17
Cortisone, cervical tumor induction and, 19
Cow
ovarian tumors in, 9, 44–47
uterine tumors in, 13, 27, 32–34, 60
Coypu, uterine tumors in, 31
Crab-eating monkeys, uterine tumors in, 30
Cricetus griseus, see Hamster
Cystadenocarcinomas
in domestic animals, 28, 45, 49, 53
in laboratory animals, 39
Cystadenofibromas, in laboratory animals, 38
Cystadenomas, 5, 9, 11
in domestic animals, 37, 43, 51, 52
in humans, 11–12
in laboratory animals, 38
in wild animals, 41, 42
Cystic endometrial hyperplasia, in domestic animals, 50, 52, 54–57
Cysts, ovarian, from estrogens, 8

Dachshund, uterine tumor in, 28
DBA mice, ovarian tumors in, 10, 11
DDT, teratomas in animals and, 41
Dermoid cysts
in domestic animals, 47, 56–57
in laboratory primates, 38
Dibenz[*a, h*]anthracene (DBA)
cervical tumor induction by, 17
as chemical carcinogen, 5
Diethylnitrosamine, ovarian tumor induction by, 5
Diethylstilbestrol
proliferative lesions induced by, 58
in uterine tumor induction, 14
vaginal tumor induction by, 17
Dimethylbenzanthracene (DMBA)
cervical cancer induction by, 18–19
ovarian tumor induction by, 4–11
placental tumor induction by, 16
uterine tumors induced by, 15
N,N′-Dimethyl-*N*-nitrosourea, uterine tumor induction by, 19
Dogs
ovarian tumors in
induced, 8
spontaneous, 4, 9, 49–50, 60
tumors in, classification, 27
uterine tumors in, 28–29
Domestic animals
ovarian tumors in, 43–60
uterine tumors in, 27–29, 32–34
Drosophila melanogaster, ovarian lesions in, 43
Duck, ovarian tumors in, 42, 49
Duplex uterus
in animals, 2
in humans, 2
Dutch rabbits, uterine tumors in, 35, 36
Dysgerminomas, 9
in domestic animals, 48, 49, 50, 55–56, 60

Eck fistula, 7
Elephant, uterine tumors in, 31
Elephant seal, ovarian tumor in, 41
Embryonal carcinoma, 60
Endometriosis, in monkeys, 29–30
Endometrium
cancer of, 27
in ewe, 27–28
in humans, 13
polyps of, in animals, 31
English Setter, adenocarcinoma in, 53
Enovid
cervical cancer induction by, 17
in vaginal tumor induction, 19
Epidermoid carcinoma
of endocervix, 17
in horse, 27
"Epithelial cords," 60
Equus caballus, see Horse
Estradiol-17β
in ovarian tumor of heifer, 45–46
ovarian tumorigenesis and, 9
Estrogen(s)
cervical tumor induction by, 16

Index

effect on, animal cervix, 12
ovarian tumor induction by, 8
uterine tumor induction by, 13-14, 36
in vaginal tumor induction, 19
Ewe, *see* Sheep
Eye
of guinea pig, tumor transplantation to, 36
ovarian grafts onto, 6

F_1 mice
ovarian tumors in, 6, 38–39
uterine tumors in, 15-16
F344 rats, ovarian tumors in, 39
Ferrets, ovarian tumors in, 40
Fetectomy, in placental tumor studies, 16, 20
Fibroadenomas
in laboratory animals, 31
in wild animals, 32
Fibroids, in wild and zoo mammals, 31
Fibroleiomyosarcomas, in laboratory animals, 31
Fibromas
in domestic animals, 27, 28, 34, 51
in laboratory animals, 38, 39
in wild and zoo animals, 31
Fibromyomas
in domesticated animals, 34
in humans, 13
induced, 13
in laboratory animals, 31, 40
in wild and zoo mammals, 31, 32
Fibromyxosarcoma, in domestic animals, 37–38
Fibrosarcomas
in laboratory animals, 38
of uterus, 14
in wild animals, 42
Fin whales, ovarian tumors in, 41
2-Fluorenylacetamide (FAA)
ovarian tumor induction by, 5, 7
uterine tumor induction by, 15
N,N-Fluorenyldiacetamide, uterine tumor induction in, 15
Fowl
ovarian tumors in, 4, 49
oviduct tumors in, 29
Fox Terrier ovarian tumor in, 58, 59
Friend leukemia virus, uterine tumors and, 16
Friesian heifer, ovarian tumor in, 45–46
Frog, ovarian tumors in, 42

Gallus domesticus, see Fowl
Gemsbok, uterine tumors in, 31
Genetic deletion, ovarian tumor induction by, 6
Gerbil
ovarian tumors in, 40
uterine tumors in, 31
Goat
ovarian tumors in, 37, 41
uterine tumors in, 28
Gonadotropins
elevated in pretumorous mice, 6
in ovarian tumorigenesis, 9, 12
"Granulosa cell islands" (GCI), in canine ovaries, 59, 60
Granulosa cell tumors (GCT), 12
in animals, 2, 5–7, 9, 37–60
Guinea pig
cervix of, 12
female genital tract in, 2, 3
ovarian tumors in, 5
induced, 11
spontaneous, 4, 9, 31, 39
placental tumor induction in, 16
uterine tumors in, induced, 13
Gull, ovarian tumor in, 42

Hamartomas, in wild animals, 30, 34
Hamster
female genital tract in, 3
human tumor transplantation to, 20
kidney tumors in, 8
ovarian tumors in, 5, 7
induced, 8
spontaneous, 4, 9, 39
uterine tumors in, 19
induced, 14, 15
spontaneous, 13, 31
Hare. *See also* Rabbit
ovarian tumors in, 40–43, 60
Hemangiomas
in domestic animals, 37, 49
in laboratory animals, 38
Hereford cow, placental tumor in, 34
Herpesvirus (HSV-2), vaginal tumor induction by, 19–20
Holstein cow, uterine tumor in, 34
Hormones
cervix tumor induction by, 16-17
imbalanced, in animal tumor induction, 13–14
in ovarian tumorigenesis, 8
Horse
ovarian tumors in, 9, 43–44
tumors in, classification, 27
uterine tumors in, 27
Human chorionic gonadotropin (HCG), in placental tumor induction, 16
Humans
cervical cancer in, mouse tumors compared to, 18
female genital tract in, compared to animals, 2, 3
ovarian tumors in, 9
mucinous cystadenomas, 11
tumors in, laboratory animals as hosts of, 20
Hydroxymethyl-methylbenzanthracene, ovarian tumor induction by, 4
20β-Hydroxypregn-4-en-3-one, in ovarian tumor of heifer, 45
17α-Hydroxyprogesterone, in ovarian tumor of heifer, 45
Hyena, vaginal tumor in, 32
Hypernephromas, in domestic animals, 44
Hypothalamic nucleus, destruction of, placental tumor induction by, 16

ICR/J mice, ovarian tumors in, 5, 11
IF mice, ovarian tumors in, 10
Insects, ovarian tumors in, 43
Intrauterine devices, uterine tumor induction by, 15, 20
Iodine-131, ovarian tumor induction by, 8

Jaguar, uterine tumors in, 32

Karyorrhexis, in ovarian tumors, 56
Koala, ovarian tumor in, 41

Laboratory animals
as human-tumor hosts, 20
ovarian tumors in, 2–4
placental tumor induction in, 16
uterine tumors in
induced, 13–16
spontaneous, 13, 29–31, 38–40
Labrador Retriever, ovarian tumor in, 54, 55
Larus ridibundus, see Gull
Leiomyomas, 14
in domestic animals, 27–29, 34, 37
in laboratory animals, 5, 29–31
Leiomyosarcomas, 13, 15
in domestic animals, 27, 29, 34, 36
in laboratory animals, 30, 31, 40
Leopard, uterine tumors in, 31
Lepus europaeus, see Hare
Leukemia-inducing virus, in mice, 4
Light, continuous, ovarian tumors from, 8
Lion, uterine tumors in, 31
Lipid cell tumors, in domestic animals, 48–49
Lipomas, in domesticated animals, 34
"Luteomas," in ovarian grafts, 7, 9, 10–11
Luteotropin (LH), ovarian tumorigenesis and, 7
Lymphomas, in domestic animals, 46
Lymphosarcoma, in domestic animals, 32

M520 rats, ovarian tumors in, 39
Macaca fascicularis, see Crab-eating monkeys
Macaca mulatta, uterine tumors in, 29–30
Mallard duck, ovarian tumor in, 42
Mammals, ovarian tumors in, 9
Mammary tumor virus, in mice, 4
Mare, uterine tumors in, 27
Marmosets
herpes infections of, 19

Marmosets [*cont.*]
  uterine tumors in, 30
Masculinization, in heifer with ovarian tumor, 45–46
Mastomys, ovarian tumors in, 40
Medroxyprogesterone, in carcinogen tumor induction, 15
Meriones sp., uterine tumors in, 31
Mesenchymal mixed tumors, in laboratory animals, 31
Mesotheliomas, uterine, 14
Mesuprine, ovarian tumor induction by, 5
Metastases, of uterine tumors, 33–36
Methotrexate, tumor transplant inhibition by, 20
3-Methylcholanthrene
  cervical tumor induction by, 18
  ovarian tumor induction by, 5
  uterine tumor induction by, 14–15
Methylthiouracil
  cervical tumor induction and, 19
  ovarian tumor induction by, 8
Mice
  cervical tumors in, 18
    induced, 16–17
  cervix of, 12
  female genital tract in, 2, 3
  ovarian tumors in
    induced, 2, 4–9
    metastatic, 11
    spontaneous, 2–4, 38–39
  uterine tumors in, 13, 30
  vaginal and cervical epithelium of, 13
  vaginal tumors in, induced, 17
101 mice, ovarian tumors in, 3
129 mice, uterine tumors in, 13
MIH Black Rats, uterine tumors of, 15
Mink, uterine tumors in, 31
Mirounga leonina, see Elephant seal
Mixed mesodermal tumors, in domestic animals, 46
Moloney's mouse sarcoma virus, placental tumor induction by, 16
Monkeys
  herpes infections in, 19
  ovarian tumors in, spontaneous, 4, 9, 38
  uterine tumors in
    induced, 14
    spontaneous, 13, 29–30
Montbéliard cow, placental tumor in, 34
Muscovy duck, ovarian tumor in, 49
Myomas
  in laboratory animals, 31, 37
  in wild and zoo mammals, 31
Myosarcomas, in laboratory animals, 37

New Zealand mice, ovarian tumors in, 6, 38
Norethandrolone, in uterine tumor induction, 15
Norethinodrone, ovarian tumor induction by, 8
Norethynodrel
  ovarian tumor induction by, 8
  uterine tumor induction by, 14
19-Norprogesterone, ovarian tumor induction by, 8
"Nude" gene, in mice, ovarian tumors and, 6
"Nude" mice, human tumor transplantation to, 20
Nylghaie, uterine tumors in, 31

"Old Buffalo" mice, uterine tumors in, 13
OM rats, ovarian tumors in, 39
Oocytes
  in mouse, 2
    tumorigenesis and, 12, 38–39
Oryctolagus cuniculus, see Rabbit
Ovarian fragmentation, uterine tumor induction by, 14
Ovarian tumors
  animal models for, 1–25
  in domesticated animals, 37–38, 43–60
  in humans, 9
  induction of, in mice, 2, 4–9
  in laboratory animals, spontaneous, 2–4
  pathology and histogenesis of, 9–11
  spontaneous, 37–60
Ovary(ies)
  in animals, 2, 3
  intrasplenic grafting of, to a castrate, tumors from, 6–7
  spontaneous tumors of, 26–65
  as tumor model, 2–9
Oviduct
  in animals, 2
  of hens, tumors of, 49, 60
Ovis aries, see Sheep
Ox, tumors in, classification, 27

Pan troglodytes, see Chimpanzees
Pancreas, ovarian transplantation to, tumors from, 7
Papanicolaou smears, of dog ascitic fluid, 53
Papillary carcinomas, in domestic animals, 57–58
Papillomas
  in domestic animals, 50–51
  in wild animals, 41
Parabiosis, with castrate, in mice, ovarian tumors from, 7
Passeriformes, in wild animals, 42
Pekin duck, ovarian tumor in, 49
Pelican, ovarian tumor in, 42
Penis
  anatomy of, in animals, 2
  epidermoid carcinoma of, in horse, 27
  herpes infection of, in monkeys, 20
Percheron mare, ovarian tumor in, 43
Persian cat
  ovarian tumor in, 49
  uterine tumor in, 28, 29
Peruvian wild ass, ovarian tumor in, 43–44
Phascolarctos cinereus, see Koala
Phasianus colchicus, see Pheasant
Pheasant, ovarian tumors in, 42
Pig, tumors in, classification, 27
Pituitary growth hormone, uterine tumor induction by, 14
Pituitary tumor, transplantation of, ovarian tumorigenesis in, 7
Placental tumors
  induced, 16
  spontaneous, 34
PM mice, uterine tumors in, 13
Pointer, ovarian tumor in, 57
Polyethylene glycol, *see* Carbowax 1000
Pony, ovarian tumor in, 44, 45
Poodle (miniature), ovarian tumor in, 58
Porcupines, uterine tumors in, 31
Primates, uterine tumors in, 29–30, 38
Progestational agents, in ovarian tumorigenesis, 8
Progesterone
  in cervical cancer induction, 18
  murine ovarian tumors and, 5
  in ovarian tumor of heifer, 45
  ovarian tumor induction by, 8
  in uterine tumor induction, 14
  in vaginal tumor induction, 19
Pyometra
  in animal uteri, 13
  in dog, 28
  in domestic animals, 50, 52, 54–57
  from estrogens, 8
  in laboratory animals, 31
Pyoovarium, from estrogens, 8

Quarter Horse, ovarian tumors in, 43

RIII mice, ovarian tumors in, 6
Rabbit
  female genital tract in, 2, 3
  ovarian tumors in, 4, 5, 60
    induced, 7
  uterine tumors in, 32
    in edible animal, 36
    induced, 14
    spontaneous, 13, 27, 34–37
Racehorse mare, ovarian tumor in, 44
Rana sp., *see* Frog
Rat
  cervix of, 12
    tumors of, 18
  female genital tract in, 2, 3, 39
  ovarian tumors in
    induced, 4–9
    spontaneous, 39
  uterine tumors in
    induced, 14
    spontaneous, 13

Index

Rauscher leukemia virus, uterine tumors and, 16
Registry of Tumors in the Lower Animals (RTLA), 27
Rhesus monkeys
  herpes, infections of, 19
  uterine tumors in, 30
Rodents, ovarian tumors in, spontaneous, 9
Sable antelope, uterine tumors in, 31
Saguinus (*Oepomidas*) *oedipus, see* Marmoset
Saimiri sciurea, see Squirrel monkey
Sarcomas
  in domestic animals, 46
  in laboratory animals, 30, 39
  of uterus, 14, 15
  in wild animals, 42
Scottish terrier, ovarian tumor in, 57
Seal
  ovarian tumors in, 41
  uterine tumor in, 32
Seminomas
  in domestic animals, 50, 55–56, 60
  in wild animals, 40
Sertoliform tubules, in rat ovary, 39, 40
Sertoliform ovarian tumors, in domestic animals, 46, 49, 50, 53-55, 58–60
Sheep
  ovarian tumors in, 9, 37
  tumors in, classification, 27
  uterine tumors in, 27–28
Simplex uterus, 2
Smegma
  human, vaginal tumors and, 17
  penile epidermoid carcinoma in horse and, 27
Soteronol, ovarian tumor induction by, 5
Sow
  ovarian tumors in, 37–38
  uterine tumors in, 28
Spaying, of animals, tumor incidence and, 27
Spleen, ovarian transplantation to, tumors from, 6–7, 9
Squamous cell carcinoma(s)
  in domestic animals, 29, 37
  in laboratory animals, 30, 31
  of uterus, 15
  in wild animals, 32
Squamous epithelium, in female genital tract, 2, 3
Squamous metaplasia, in fowl, 29
Squirrel
  ovarian tumors in, 41
  uterine tumors in, 31
Squirrel monkeys
  herpes infections of, 19
  ovarian tumor in, 38
Steel (sl) genes, in mice, ovarian tumorigenesis in, 6
Stilbestrol
  ovarian tumor induction by, 8
  tumor induction by, 14
Stilbestrol-cholesterol, vaginal tumor induction by, 17
Subsurface epithelial structures (SES), in canine ovary, 58–60
Swine, wild, uterine tumors in, 31

Tampons, use in carcinogen tumor induction, 15
Teratocarcinoma, 60
Teratomas, 5, 9, 11
  in domesticated animals, 37–39, 43, 46–50, 56–57, 60
  in wild animals, 40–42
Testes
  teratoma in, 11
Testicular grafts, uterine tumor induction by, 14
"Testis cords," 60
Testosterone
  cervical cancer induction by, 17, 19
  ovarian tumor induction by, 8, 9
  in uterine tumor induction, 14
Theca cell tumors
  in domestic animals, 49
  in rats, 8
Thecomas
  in domestic animals, 45
  in laboratory animals, 39
  in monkey, 38
Thread, in cervical and vaginal tumor induction, 17–19, 20
Thymectomy, ovarian tumor induction by, 6
Thyroid hormone, effects on ovarian tumorigenesis, 8
L-Thyroxine, cervical tumor induction and, 19
Toxemia of pregnancy, uterine tumors and, 36
Transplantation
  ovarian tumorigenesis by, 5–6
  of uterine tumors, 36
Triethylene melamine, ovarian tumor induction by, 5
Trimethylbenzanthracene, ovarian tumor induction by, 4–5
Tubular adenomas, ovarian, induced, 10
Tumors
  ovarian, *see* Ovarian tumors
  uterine, *see* Uterine tumors
Urethane, ovarian tumor induction by, 5, 11, 12
Uterine tumors
  animal models for, 1–25
  spontaneous, 27–37
Uterus
  in animals, 2
  metaplasia of, from estrogens, 8
  prenatal changes in, 12
  spontaneous tumors of, 26–65
  as tumor model, 12–16

Vagina
  animal models for tumors of, 16
  epidermoid carcinoma of, 27
  perinatal changes in, 12
Vasoligation, of ovary, tumor induction by, 6
Vinyl copolymer, uterine tumor induction by, 15
Viruses
  placental tumor induction by, 16
  uterine tumor induction by, 15-16, 19, 20
Vulva
  animal models for tumors of, 16
  epidermoid carcinoma of, 27
  tumors of, in animals, 13

W genes, in mice, ovarian tumorigenesis in, 6
Wn rats, ovarian tumors in, 39
Whale
  ovarian tumors in, 41
  uterine tumor in, 32
Wild animals
  ovarian tumors in, 40–43
  uterine tumors in, 31–34
Wistar rats, in laboratory animals, 39

X rays
  cervical tumor induction and, 19
  ovarian tumor induction by, 4
  uterine tumor induction by, 15, 20

Yak, uterine tumors in, 31

Zebu cattle, ovarian tumors in, 46–49, 60
Zoo animals
  ovarian tumors in, 40–43
  uterine tumors in, 31–32